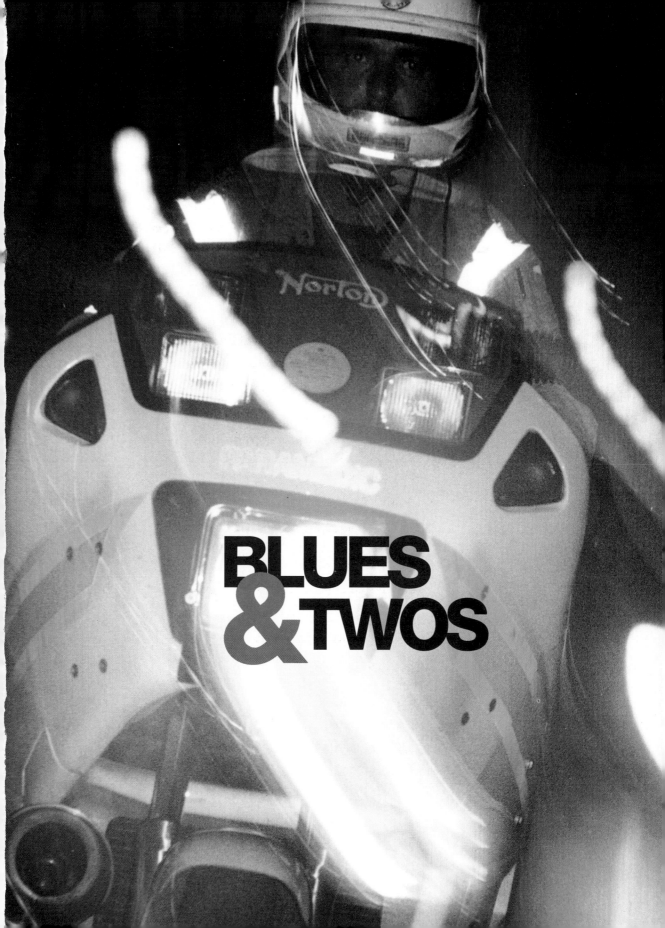

Also by Ivan Rendall

FLYERS: THE SPIRIT OF KITTY HAWK

REACHING FOR THE SKIES:
A HISTORY OF MANNED FLIGHT

THE POWER AND THE GLORY:
A CENTURY OF MOTOR RACING

THE CHEQUERED FLAG:
100 YEARS OF MOTOR RACING

AYRTON SENNA: A TRIBUTE

Cover photograph: London paramedic Allan
Norman on his way to a casualty by motorcycle.
Allan's work as the paramedic with the
Helicopter Emergency Service featured in the
Blues and Twos pilot programme, 'Medevac',
then in 'Solo One', when he retrained on
motorcycles.

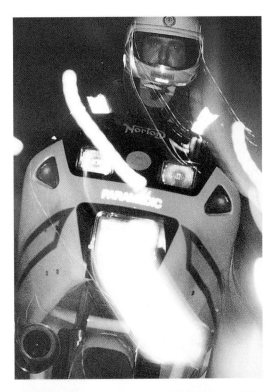

BLUES
&TWOS
IVAN RENDALL

LITTLE, BROWN AND COMPANY

A *Little, Brown* Book

First published in Great Britain by Little, Brown and Company 1995

Copyright © Ivan Rendall, Carlton Television Limited, Zenith North Ltd 1995

The moral right of the author has been asserted.

A CIP catalogue record for this book
is available from the British Library.

Typeset in Sabon by M Rules
Printed in Italy

Little, Brown and Company (UK)
Brettenham House
Lancaster Place
London WC2E 7EN

Pictures were supplied or reproduced by kind permission of the following: Carlton
Television: i, iii, 6, 7, 14, 22, 23, 50, 51, 190, 214; courtesy Express Newspapers:
157; Glasgow Herald: 128; H.E.M.S.: 11; Hulton Deutsch Collection: 34, 35, 48,
92, 93, 162; Impact Photos: 2, 4, 106; Magnum/David Hurn: 62–3; Mary Evans
Picture Library: 28, 32, 42; Mary Evans Picture Library/Bruce Castle Museum: 37;
Metropolitan Police Museum: 33 above, 45; Museum of the Order of St John: 39,
40, 41; Press Association: 160, 161; Popperfoto: 33 below, 49, 56, 58, 66, 71, 88;
Popperfoto/Reuter: 184, 188, 191; Rex Features: 5, 10, 15, 59, 74–5, 79, 82, 109,
112, 118, 120, 121, 123, 134–5, 138, 139, 142, 150, 158, 165, 166, 169, 174,
175, 178, 180, 182, 186, 187, 202, 204, 210, 211, 212; Royal National Lifeboat
Institution: 30, 31, 206, 207, 208; Scunthorpe Evening Telegraph: 65, 67; Sygma:
3, 102, 126, 127, 179, 197, 198, 200; Topham Picture Source: 18, 46, 78, 95,
101, 107, 114, 115, 143, 148, 149, 152, 164, 194, 196, 209.

CONTENTS

For all the men and women who work
in the emergency and rescue services.

INTRODUCTION

Rarely does a television or radio news bulletin go by without a disaster being reported somewhere in Britain or around the world. A train crash, a motorway pile-up, a shooting incident, a terrorist bomb, a ship foundering in high seas, climbers lost in the mountains, an air crash, a house fire – are all news. And at the heart of every story is the work of the emergency services. Disasters don't only happen on television; hardly a day goes by, especially living in a large city, without seeing the flashing blue lights and hearing the wailing two-tone sirens of police cars, fire appliances or ambulances on their way to the thousands of personal disasters which never make the news.

In today's world it is almost impossible not to be aware of the work of the emergency services, yet the real-life rescuers are largely anonymous: men and women in fluorescent jackets calmly reassuring people in distress and taking the injured away to safety. Occasionally there may be a short sound bite from one of them on the news to explain what happened, but even if we hear their names we rarely remember them. And yet, individually and collectively, it is impossible not to admire them. In a world conspicuously free of great heroic figures, they have become the popular heroes of

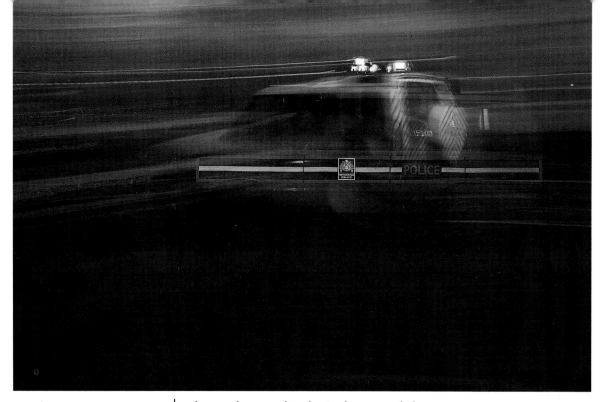

A Police Range Rover on its way to an emergency: the expression 'blues and twos' was coined by police drivers in the 1960s to describe driving to an incident with blue lights and sirens on over the radio.

the modern, technological age, and their quiet competence, caring determination and simple courage have become part of popular culture.

Stories of saving life are gripping stuff, and the action-packed, caring world of the emergency services has been explored from every angle by the main provider of popular culture – television. Documentary series such as ITV's *Blues and Twos* and feature programmes such as the BBC's *999* attract huge audiences, and the same themes of modern reality, human frailty and individual resourcefulness have become the basis of some of the most popular drama series, both home produced and imported from America, for over thirty years: *Dixon of Dock Green, Emergency Ward Ten, Z Cars, The Bill, London's Burning, Hill Street Blues, Casualty, ER,* and many more. Their huge fascination, whether they are 'reality' programmes or drama, has turned them into a major part of every TV station's schedule.

There are people who are critical of the number of such programmes, and of the trend towards more and more reality which some dismiss as mere 'ambulance chasing'. The more positive explanation is that they have simply evolved as part of a natural balance in the television diet which both viewers and broadcasters need. Television is a window on the world, and it can be a very dark and troubled world at times; uplifting stories of selflessness, especially when they are patently true, help to reassure us that the world is also still a humane place.

When a bomb blew apart the United States Federal Government building in Oklahoma City in April 1995, President Bill Clinton praised the rescue workers as all politicians do when they visit the scene of a disaster. His speech was predictable, and no less genuine and heartfelt for that, but his wife Hillary went further. Asked to address herself specifically to the many children who had been disturbed and upset by the thought that there were such evil people in American society, she pointed out that, while the reality is that there are exceptionally evil people in the world, there are also exceptionally good people. As she made her speech she was pointing to the men and women of the rescue services whom the same children had seen in the very same television pictures of the carnage, pulling survivors from the rubble and continuing to search the dangerously unstable building for any sign of life.

Hillary Clinton was right. From whatever service they come, whether paramedics, police officers, fire fighters, ambulancemen

The triumph and tragedy of rescue work: an Oklahoma fireman, Chris Fields, cradles a young girl, Baylee Almon, taken alive from the wreckage of the Federal Government Building in Oklahoma City which was blown apart by a terrorist car bomb in April 1995. Baylee died later the same day.

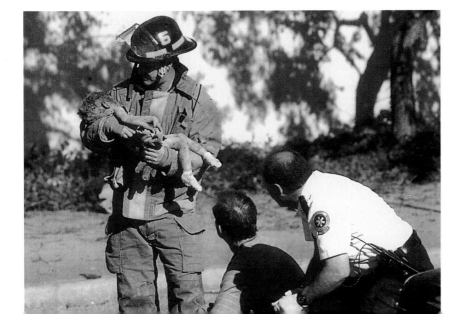

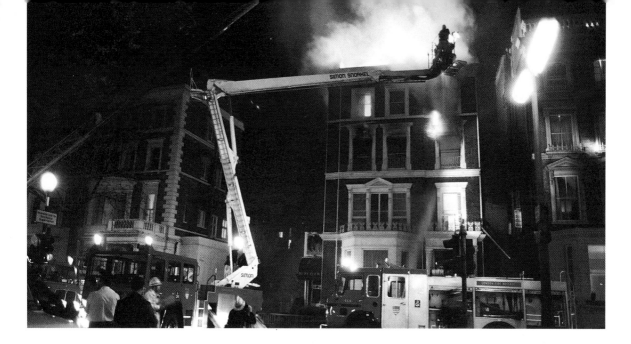

London's burning: London firemen dousing a house fire; the capital's fire brigade receives over 500 calls a day, the busiest station is in Soho.

and women, lifeboatmen, helicopter rescue pilots and winchmen, or Army bomb disposal officers, the members of the rescue services have a real stature in modern societies. They are part of popular culture, but at the same time they have retained – and this is doubtless part of their attraction – strong traditional values of service in a precarious world.

For most of history, the only disasters were natural – floods, fires, storms, earthquakes, typhoons, tidal waves, hurricanes, and volcanoes. In the last 200 years, technology, while improving the quality of life in many respects, has also added to the potential for disaster: nuclear power stations, high-rise buildings, high-speed motorways, ever faster and more crowded transport systems to cross the oceans and continents by land, sea and air. We are constantly challenging the natural world with more technological wizardry, improving life while putting ourselves at ever-greater risk when that technology fails, as history demonstrates it inevitably will. When things do go wrong with modern technology, the results are both spectacular and deadly: nuclear power stations and chemical factories do explode, high-rise buildings do collapse or catch fire, aircraft do crash, car ferries do overturn, underground trains

4

do run out of control, explosions do happen in coal mines and their thousand-foot lift shafts do fail. In the last twenty-five years, terrorists have added another, chilling, layer of potential for disaster by planting bombs and poisonous gas canisters deliberately designed to kill and maim.

Technology has made the world more dangerous but, paradoxically, it has also made it safer. To see a modern helicopter, a marvel of science and technology, hover serenely over a storm-tossed, sinking ship, gently winching a crew member to safety, is to watch one of the triumphs of human ingenuity over the forces of nature. Self-righting lifeboats, thermal-imaging cameras to find victims buried under rubble, ambulances equipped with oxygen and defibrillators to restart the heart after a heart attack, have all increased our chances of survival if we do get into trouble and today we expect to be saved from all kinds of difficulties, from climbing on an icy mountain without the correct equipment, to a house fire caused by a lighted cigarette, to a capsized ferry in a freezing sea.

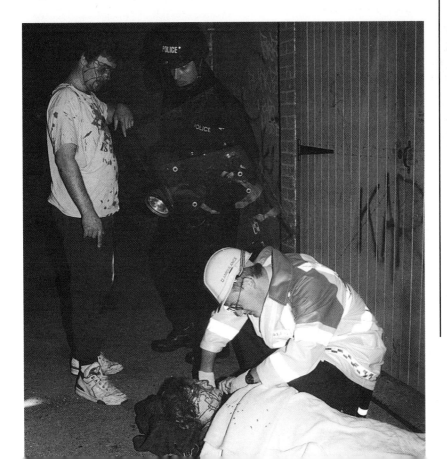

Modern popular heroes: a police officer and an ambulance officer deal with a stabbing during a riot in Oxford in 1991.

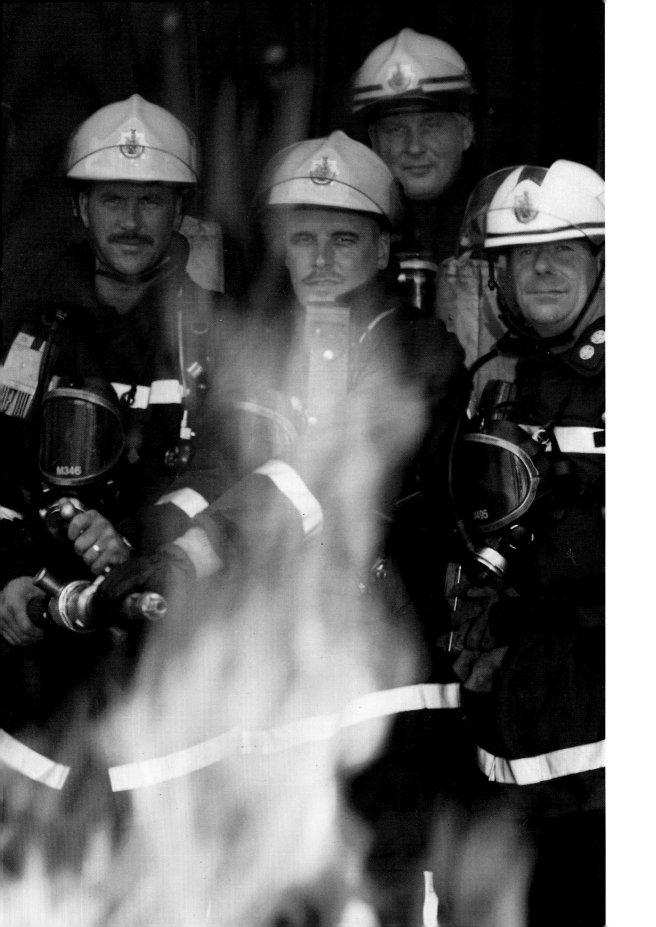

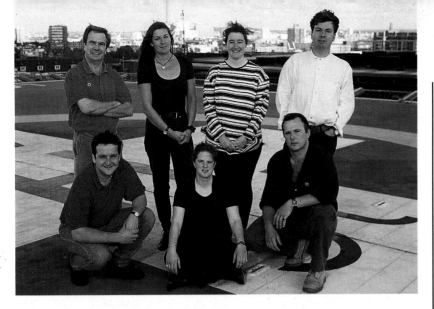

Equally, when modern weather forecasting fails, or the forces of nature are just too unpredictable and awesome to cope with, we look to the emergency services for help. The list is never ending: the Great Storm of 1987, the San Francisco earthquake of 1989, the Bengal cyclone and floods of 1991, the Los Angeles earthquake and fire of 1993, the Mississippi floods the same year, the Sydney fires in 1994 and the Kobe earthquake in 1995.

Technology does save lives, but technology does not do anything without people. *Blues and Twos* is about people. Its format is simple: it tells the stories of people who find themselves at the centre of disasters, both the victims who need saving and those who do the saving. The title is taken from emergency service radio jargon for driving with blue lights flashing and two-tone sirens wailing and it reflects the central theme behind the series: the reality of what happens in disasters. Both the television series and this book are about the people whose job is to keep their heads in often very difficult circumstances, and who sometimes put their own lives in jeopardy in order to save others.

It is the story of some very special people.

Ivan Rendall
Kings Green, Worcester
May 1995

Left: Blues and Twos production team, from left to right, standing: John Pettman (Series Producer), Sarah Ann Cockroft (Associate Producer), Rachel Goodwin (Researcher), Andrew Fettis (Director, Series 1); kneeling: Tom Brisley (Director, Series 2), Alison Grade (Production Manager), Mark Jackson (mini-camera specialist).

Opposite: The Manchester County Fire Service is one of the busiest in the country outside London, attending 66,000 incidents a year, from which 250 lives are saved. The crew who featured in *Blues and Twos* are from left to right: Martin Sykes, Steve Brooks, Bob Curtis, Mick Collins.

Chapter One

BLUES AND TWOS –
THE INSIDE STORY

Some time early in the morning of Saturday 25 April 1993, a group of IRA terrorists parked a blue tipper lorry containing a bomb in Bishopsgate outside the London headquarters of the Hong Kong & Shanghai Bank. It was just fifty yards from the fifty-two-storey NatWest tower, the second tallest building in the City of London and a symbol of its importance as an international financial centre. A little further away was the Commercial Union Insurance building; just round the corner was the Baltic Exchange, which had been demolished by an IRA bomb just over a year previously, and a few minutes' walk away was the Lloyd's insurance building, the Bank of England and the Stock Exchange.

The Bishopsgate bomb was designed to show that the IRA was in no mood to give up its campaign. It was one of the largest bombs the IRA had managed to plant on the mainland and they had placed it right at the economic heart of the country with perfect timing. That weekend, hundreds of delegates had arrived in the City for the annual meeting of the European Bank for Reconstruction and Development. Also on that Saturday, as part of continuing and very tentative moves towards peace in Ireland, the parents of two small boys killed in a Warrington shopping precinct

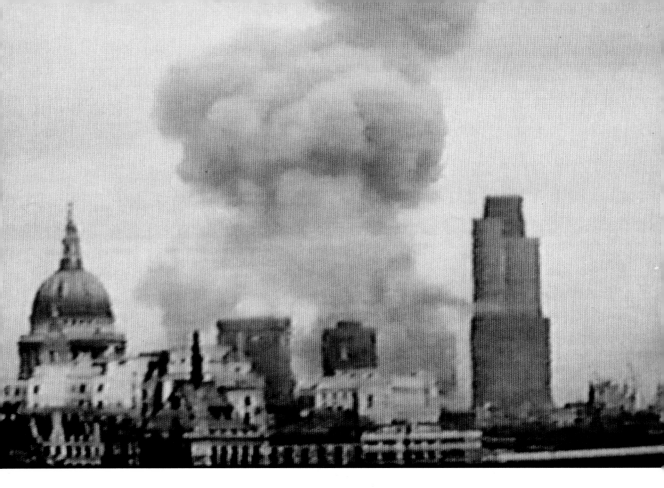

Bishopsgate bomb, 24 April 1993: in a scene reminiscent of the Blitz, one of the largest bombs the IRA ever planted on the mainland explodes close to St Paul's Cathedral in smoke; the blast was felt across the city.

a month previously by an IRA bomb in a litter bin were in Dublin in support of peace.

The first warning was phoned to the police at 9.17a.m. using an established code. There were eight calls in all, designed to confuse London's emergency services as they were put on alert. Police combed the area around Bishopsgate, clearing pedestrians from the streets and identifying likely vehicles. It was the weekend and though the buildings were largely unoccupied, some people were working in offices and there was maintenance work going on. Police warned security guards in each building of the bomb threat and advised them to take everybody inside to safety, preferably below street level. In the Hong Kong & Shanghai bank, secretaries and maintenance workers joked as they were ushered into the basement, believing it was simply a hoax.

In Whitechapel, barely a mile away from Bishopsgate, is the London Hospital. It is one of the City's major hospitals and home to London's Helicopter Emergency Medical Service (HEMS) which operates a bright orange helicopter ambulance from a helipad on the roof. The HEMS pilots are drawn largely from the armed forces and they are cleared to land anywhere in London – in the street, on top of a building or any open space which is big enough to take the helicopter. HEMS is only called to emergencies which need urgent attention, the principal advantage of a helicopter ambulance being that it can transport a doctor with a high level of skill in emergency medicine to a seriously injured person much more quickly than by picking up the same patient in a road ambulance and driving to hospital. Emergency medical teams call the first hour after an accident 'the golden hour', and treatment in that hour hugely increases the patient's chances of survival. The HEMS doctor is backed up by a specially trained paramedic; they work as a team using a wide range of life-saving equipment which it would be impossible to carry in every ambulance. Once the patient has been stabilised,

HEMS attending a Road Traffic Accident in London; in six years, the helicopter ambulance has attended 6,247 incidents, over half of them traffic accidents, has landed six times in Piccadilly Circus and fifteen times in Trafalgar Square.

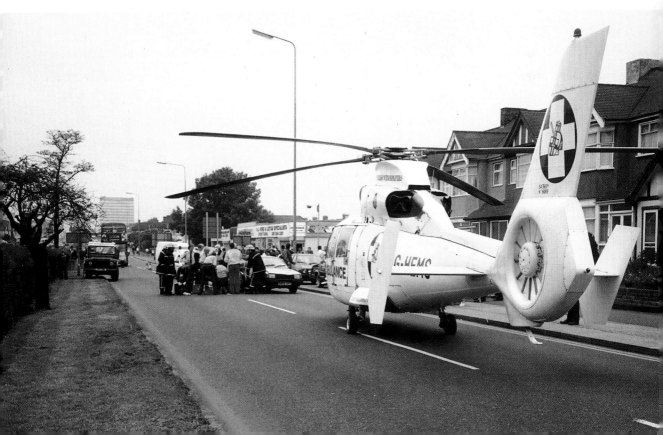

the helicopter can then take them wherever the best treatment is: a hospital with a specialist burns unit, for example, or a spinal injury unit.

That Saturday morning, the duty paramedic was Allan Norman and the doctor was Karen Heath, a young Army doctor on attachment to the National Health Service. At 9.30a.m. they were called to an elderly lady who had been run over by a truck in Fulham and was trapped under it. Minutes after taking off, the two pilots, Richard Shuttleworth and Ian Field, landed on the lawn of a block of flats, leaving Karen and Allan only the last few hundred yards to run to the scene of the accident in Lillie Road. When they got there, they found that the front wheels of the truck had gone right over the woman and she had multiple injuries to her legs and the lower part of her body. By 10 o'clock they were well on the way to stabilising their patient and getting her out from under the truck, but instead of flying her out, they decided to take her by road to the Charing Cross Hospital which was nearby. Karen and Allan went with the patient in the ambulance, leaving Richard and Ian free to fly to the Battersea heliport to refuel. They arranged to meet up again at a children's playground in a park in Lillie Road.

With HEMS that day was a television cameraman. He was working for Zenith North, an independent television production company which had chosen that weekend to shoot a pilot programme for a new series about the work of the emergency services, *Blues and Twos*. It had been commissioned by London's ITV company, Carlton Television. Instead of a production team following the main characters, there was just one cameraman. The technique was true 'fly on the wall' documentary making, using a whole series of micro-technology cameras and sound systems positioned as discreetly as possible to record everything that was going on during a rescue, as well as the conventional television camera. The idea was to eavesdrop on the action from as many angles as possible, from as close as possible. The mini-cameras were fitted throughout the helicopter showing the pilots at their controls and Karen and Allan in the cabin behind where the patient is carried. Karen even had a tiny camera sewn into the front of her flying overalls and a tiny video recorder in her pocket so that everything she did was filmed in close-up.

The other members of the television team were filming at the two other places concerned with controlling the movements of the helicopter: the London Ambulance Service main control room in Waterloo where all the 999 calls come in, and the HEMS control room on top of the London Hospital. In that way, the whole sequence of events leading up to a rescue, from the 999 call being received to the patient being delivered to the hospital, could be shown in sequence and in detail, including the exchanges over the telephone and radio networks.

At Waterloo, the producer, John Pettman, and associate producer, Sarah Ann Cockroft, were covering the incoming 999 calls, showing the controllers sifting them, then deciding what to do in each case and whether to send the helicopter. If it was to be sent, then the orders were relayed to the HEMS control room at the London Hospital where two more members of the production team were waiting: the director, Andrew Fettis, and the researcher, Rachel Goodwin. They had rigged the control room with mini-cameras and sound systems to show the HEMS controller Mike Griffiths at work, recording all his radio conversations with the pilots.

Everybody in the emergency services was aware of the bomb threat. The police had put London Ambulance HQ and all the major hospitals on standby as soon as the warning came through. Following the alert, the mood in the Waterloo control room changed slightly, but only slightly, to an air of expectancy. There were still 'routine' 999 calls coming in from across the capital,

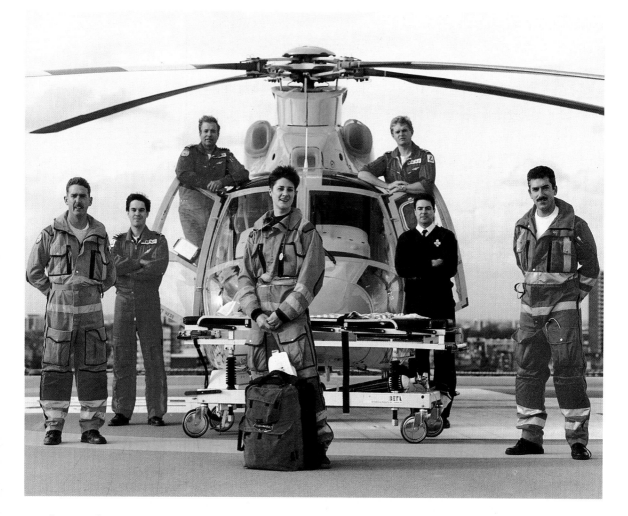

London's Helicopter Emergency Medical Service. The HEMS team, 24 April 1993: from left to right, Allan Norman, paramedic, Dave Gurney, pilot, Richard Shuttleworth, pilot, Major (Dr) Karen Heath, doctor, Ian Field, pilot, Mark Griffiths, controller and Les Bernard, paramedic. On average the helicopter is called out three times a day; the highest ever number of call-outs in a day was nine. Over half the calls are to Road Traffic Accidents (RTAs). The priority is to minimise the effects of serious injury. The helicopter can land anywhere in London: the pilots find busy road junctions the most difficult and among the most interesting are Oxford Circus, Piccadilly Circus and Trafalgar Square. It is impossible to say how many lives have been saved by HEMS directly, but informed opinion believes it to be around twelve a year.

and the warning might still turn out to be a hoax, so it was business as usual as the controllers went about their duties in the familiar, hushed tones.

At 10.25a.m., a ton of fertiliser was detonated in the back of the blue tipper lorry. It blew a forty-foot crater in the road and the explosion was heard across most of London; the lorry's engine finished up over fifty yards away. People felt the shock wave all around the City. In the streets, in shops and hotels, windows smashed and shelves emptied as a result of the physical impact of the explosion. In the immediate area around Bishopsgate, acres of glass from the tall buildings cascaded into the streets. The police had cleared most of them, so mercifully there were few people underneath the falling shards. In the basement of the Hong Kong & Shanghai Bank, the people were still joking as the bomb went off. Even below street level they were blown off their feet while above them the ceiling collapsed. Seconds later clouds of black smoke started filling the basement. Peter Redman, a London

A fireman in Bishopsgate after the explosion: the emergency services were on alert when the bomb went off and arrived on the scene despite the threat of a second bomb.

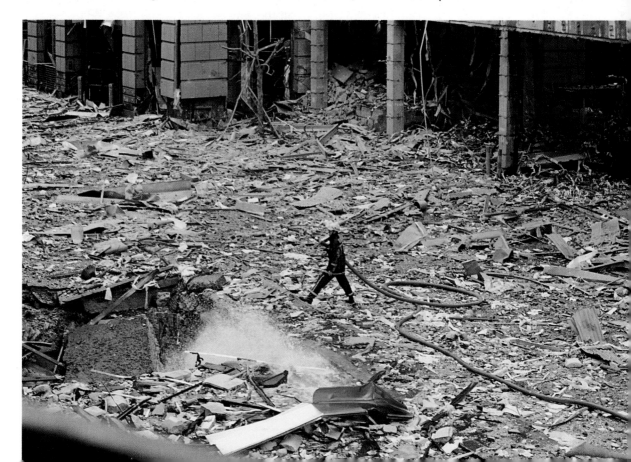

Ambulance paramedic on a motorcycle, was blown off and landed in the gutter, winded.

When the shock wave hit the HEMS control room at the London Hospital, it caused electronic interference: Mark Griffiths' radio went dead and the picture of him on the television monitor went to fuzzy black and white lines. In the kitchen, Andrew Fettis was just opening a yoghurt for breakfast when the lights went out. He went to the control room and asked Mark what had happened, assuming it was a power cut. Then they heard the explosion: the glass flexed in the window frames, kitchen utensils rattled and bottles shuddered on shelves and the whole building shook.

'What's that?' asked one of the firemen who was standing by for the return of the helicopter.

'It's a bomb, a bloody great bomb,' said Mark, just as his radio started to function again and his picture reappeared on the television monitor.

Andrew Fettis headed for the landing pad, instinctively grabbing a small video camera on the way. As he reached the railings, he saw the top of a dark, dirty-brown mushroom cloud billowing up between the skyscrapers. He turned on the camera and filmed it, and as he did so, it grew larger and larger, violently at first, before dispersing and drifting over the City.

At London Ambulance HQ, John Pettman and Sarah Cockroft also heard the bomb go off. They had been half expecting it but both of them were astonished by the cool-headed way everybody responded to the first reports that it had exploded. With complete calm, the supervisors brought a separate desk into operation, with its own dedicated radio channel and telephone lines solely to coordinate calls relating to the bomb incident. The 999 controllers were inundated with calls, both from members of the public and over the radio from ambulance crews round the city who had heard the bomb go off and were asking for instructions where to go. It was assumed that there would be a great many very serious casualties, so hospitals were put on red alert and off-duty staff and surgeons called in.

There had been warnings of a second bomb which might be timed to go off just as the rescue services arrived to treat casualties, so the police had cordoned off a huge area and advised people in the buildings to stay where they were. The streets inside the cordon were strewn with broken glass and rubble. At the Hong Kong & Shanghai Bank people lay on the floor covered in debris from the fallen ceiling. No one in the basement was badly hurt, but two of the security men who had still been searching the building as the bomb went off were badly injured.

At the Battersea heliport, Richard and Ian had refuelled the helicopter and they were ready to take off as the news came over the radio. They lifted off immediately and headed towards Fulham to collect Karen, Allan and the cameraman who were still at the Charing Cross Hospital. Immediately they were airborne again, they flew towards the City. As they approached they could see the devastation, smoke still rising over tall glass buildings which were completely gutted. Richard decided that it would be too dangerous to land in the street as the sound of the helicopter's engines and the downwash from the rotor blades would almost certainly bring more glass crashing down causing even more casualties, including rescue workers who were already gathering below. Instead he flew straight back to the London Hospital helipad. Karen and Allan had already decided they would go to the scene of the explosion by road, so once they had landed, they grabbed new medical supplies, then drove to a rendezvous point just outside the police cordon. The cameraman collected fresh batteries and new videotapes and went with them.

At the rendezvous they waited for instructions. The police had cleared the streets and inside their cordon the City was deserted.

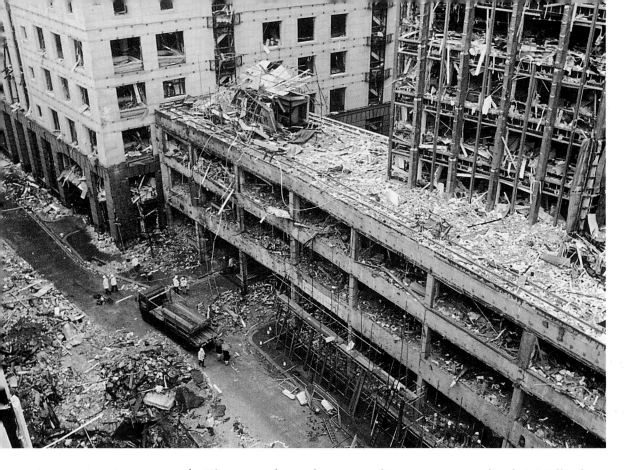

Clearing up at the Hong Kong & Shanghai Bank building in Bishopsgate; the crater in the road (left foreground) marks the spot where the lorry bomb was parked.

The worst fears about casualties were not realised: initially there were no reports of any deaths and the first estimate of people injured was forty, most of whom were already on their way to hospital. The main task now was to search the streets and buildings for other injured people, and possibly for bodies. A policeman took Karen and Allan through the eerie streets in single file, walking in the middle of the road to avoid any falling glass. There was silence, except for the sound of dozens of fire alarms. It was an extraordinary sight inside the police cordon, deserted streets covered by a carpet of glass fragments. They searched for about an hour but found nobody and they were eventually released to go back on standby at the London Hospital.

Police, fire and ambulance officers continued to search through the afternoon. The people sheltering in their buildings were advised to stay there for several hours and were taken out only once the police had checked that there were no more bombs. In mid-afternoon, they found the body of Edward Henty, a thirty-four-year-old freelance photographer, who was buried under rubble near the Hong Kong & Shanghai Bank. He had heard of the possibility of a bomb and driven to the City shortly before it exploded; he was the only fatality.

Any death is tragic, but considering the short time available to clear the streets, the deliberately confusing nature of the warnings and the possibility of a second bomb, it was a huge testimony to the work of the emergency services that only one person died. Without their prompt actions the death toll would undoubtedly have been much higher. The number of injured finally rose to fifty-one, but they had all been taken to hospital quickly.

The emergency services' plans for a major incident had been put into effect immediately and they had worked. From the moment the bomb went off until the incident was over, the calm atmosphere in the London Ambulance control room barely changed: heads stayed bent over microphones and computer screens; flashing lights denoting emergencies were answered in order; conversation stayed muted; telephone calls were brief and to the point.

The idea behind *Blues and Twos* – what the pilot programme was designed to show – was precisely that professionalism in the most realistic circumstances possible. It was devised as a close-up view of the work of the emergency services from the inside, literally working alongside them in a major disaster. Above all, the idea was to show the reality of people whose working lives are spent in dangerous circumstances, and to do so without sanitising what they actually do by using the artifice of reconstruction. By making it real, the audience could see them for the very special kind of people they are, not through drama or by being told that they are special, but by seeing them actually making decisions – some life and death – under the pressure of stressful situations. In that sense, the day of the Bishopsgate bomb was a perfect illustration of what the series was trying to do.

During the afternoon Karen and Allan went on several other emergency missions in London, none of which made the news, but all of which involved treatment of major injuries on the spot. After a twelve-hour shift they went off duty, then came back on Sunday morning for another shift. Just as impressive were the controllers, the ambulancemen and women who called as in they calmly headed for the disaster, not knowing what to expect, except the possibility of a second bomb. If anything proved that a television series which showed that professionalism in real close-up would be worthwhile, then the events of that Saturday morning did.

The footage that the *Blues and Twos* team had shot was a unique record of the event. It was intended for a documentary but there was an immediate demand for it from television news editors in Britain and abroad. Carlton TV released it to ITV and BBC and to agencies who sent it round the world, particularly Andrew Fettis's shot of the smoke rising over the city and the clip of Mark Griffiths when the mini-camera went dead as the bomb went off; they were repeated on every bulletin. During the night, Mark Griffiths was woken by a phone call from his aunt in Australia who had seen him on the news, then disappear as the screen went dead; she wanted to know that he was all right.

The footage was a journalistic coup for the whole team but particularly for Andrew, and his colleagues congratulated him on it when they watched it that evening. His pictures dominated the news coverage and he was rightly proud of them, but though he could tell his family and a few friends, he could not say anything to his colleagues at work because he worked for the BBC and had been moonlighting that weekend!

The finished programme took many hours to edit, but the

technique worked; it looked very different from any previous documentary, an impressive demonstration of what mini-cameras could do. It had been commissioned by Carlton for transmission in the London area, but when the finished product was available, the ITV Network decided to put it out nationally. The title was *Medevac*, the HEMS helicopter call sign. It was broadcast in November 1993 to a 12.25 million audience, much higher than expected, and on the strength of that interest, ITV commissioned a first series of seven programmes covering the work of a variety of emergency services across the country.

What the production team had been looking for, and what they had found at HEMS, was the perfect combination of emergency services people and action which could be filmed with a closeness, intimacy almost, with the quietly spoken people who do such an extraordinary job. To capture that closeness, and show the action while still feeling involved with the individuals in the film, there had to be a relationship of trust between the producers and the people they were filming. The ground rules were simple: if ever a situation developed where the cameras could even remotely have interfered with medical treatment, the simple words 'get out' would suffice to end the filming. It was also agreed that no distressing incidents would be broadcast without the permission of the patients.

Karen Heath was the central character in *Medevac*, but before she, as a doctor, would allow cameras to be strapped to her body – literally coming between doctor and the patient – she had to be certain that such trust was not misplaced. Establishing that trust was only possible with people who had the self-confidence to give it. In the course of the weekend with HEMS, Karen went to incidents which would have been too invasive or too distressing to show on television and they were not shown. On other occasions, people were not prepared to give permission and the footage could not be used. Once it was clear that the producers would not abuse the unique access which they had been allowed, Karen and Allan forgot that the cameras were there, adding their own contribution to the 'reality' of the film by just getting on with their jobs and focusing on what they were doing.

Karen and Allan were the guinea pigs for a new kind of programme, and without their confidence in themselves and in the production team the series would never have happened. Karen returned to the Army shortly after the filming. Allan Norman, the paramedic who worked with her in Bishopsgate, left HEMS shortly afterwards to train as a motorcycle paramedic and one of the programmes in the first full series of *Blues and Twos* followed his work a year later. The title was *Solo One*, his call sign.

Brenda Blood (right) and her daughter, Estelle, in the Derbyshire Ambulance Service control room where the 999 calls come through. Estelle was one of the first 999 controllers in Britain to be trained in the '999 stay on the line' service in which controllers talk the caller through what is happening to the patient, giving first-aid advice until the paramedics arrive.

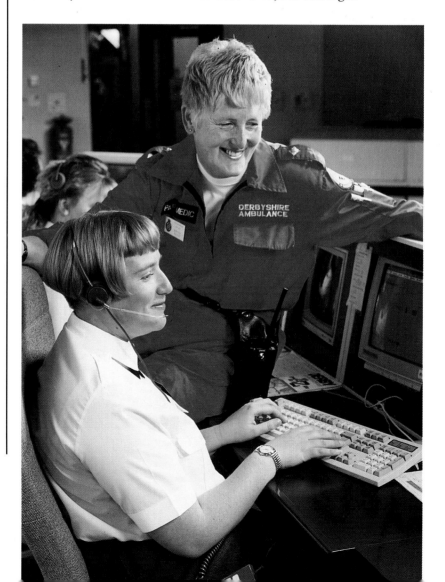

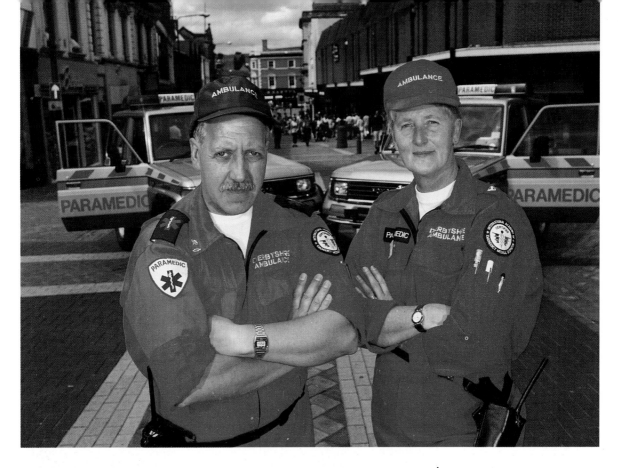

Blues and Twos was never intended to be controversial, but when the first series went out in the autumn of 1994, for a time it was attacked by television critics as being 'Ghoul on the wall' television and 'cheap'. The *Independent*'s critic called the genre 'actuality drama', and went on to say that there seemed to be 'a plague [of them] at the moment'. There seemed to be a theme running through the criticism of series 1: 'Oh no, not another series about the emergency services.'

During the seven programmes the attitude did change – it became far less dismissive, and as the audience showed its obvious interest and admiration for the people shown the negative comments dried up. By the end of the series some of the critics had seen the point, that there was a strong, positive and very humane underpinning to the subject matter and to the way it was handled. In the end, the *Observer* critic summed it up as 'humbling to watch'.

Maurice Foster and Brenda Blood, both paramedics with the Derbyshire Ambulance Service, who featured in the first programme in the first series of *Blues and Twos*.

The purpose was not only to observe the emergency services, but also to celebrate the bravery and dedication of the people in them. The declared aim of the series as set out in the original treatment was to leave the audience feeling 'Thank God there are people like that out there.' In that it was successful, for that was the overwhelming response from viewers: in a poll, 75 per cent said it was reassuring to see the efficiency of the emergency services; 1 per cent thought it in bad taste; 73 per cent said that it left them wanting to see more; 33 per cent that it was the best documentary about the emergency services; 4 per cent did not enjoy it at all.

The people in the emergency services generally loved it. Chief Inspector Malcolm Magnay of the Northumbria Police, two of whose officers had featured in the first series, said: 'Having watched the programme I was very pleased to see it reflect a different dimension to policing – the human element which is often forgotten in some of the police programmes on TV.' Stuart Ide, Chief Executive of the Derbyshire Ambulance Service, who also let the team film his paramedics at work without restriction said: 'The fact that the film crew was so unobtrusive means that what people see on their screens will be a very real reflection of the work we do.'

Chapter Two

THE HUMANITARIAN TRADITION

Britain is extraordinarily fortunate in its emergency services. The men and women of the police, fire and ambulance services are key players in the functioning of our complex, modern, but also troubled society. They work on an invisible front line, a fault line which runs through the fabric of that society, the line between danger and safety, between order and chaos, the line between coping with or succumbing to both natural and man-made disasters, the line between life and death. Their job begins when that complex society's plans for itself go wrong and we rarely meet them unless we need them desperately: lying on a busy pavement in the throes of a heart attack; having just failed to commit suicide; watching a life's work or an entire household being consumed by flames; in a police station accused of a crime or being told that a loved one has just been killed in a car accident. They are there when we need them and they provide a highly professional and caring service. In return a strong relationship of trust has developed between the emergency services and the public.

The modern emergency services have inherited a long tradition of service which has been built up over two centuries. That tradition extends beyond the 999 services to the Air/Sea Rescue services of the RAF and Royal Navy, the mountain rescue, cave rescue and above all to the Royal National Lifeboat Institution, one of the most respected rescue services anywhere in the world. Service in them appeals to characteristics which any society values: public spiritedness, boldness in adversity, practicality, the ability to improvise, personal confidence, persistence and selflessness. With their long history and their local importance, people are naturally drawn to serve in them – sons and increasingly daughters follow fathers and mothers.

It is a job, but it is also much more than a job. Lifeboatmen do not put to sea in storms, firemen do not enter burning buildings, paramedics do not clamber through wrecked trains, nor policemen face terrorists for the money. They do it for many reasons: for the camaraderie of small groups dedicated to rewarding and sometimes dangerous tasks; for the personal challenge of facing immediate and tricky situations; to test their professionalism; but above all they do it to help other people in distress, for sound and instinctively humanitarian reasons.

That humanitarian impulse is based on ideas whose origins are part of the shaping of modern Western society in the late eighteenth century during the Enlightenment, when the central idea that the life of an individual, regardless of class, was of the highest importance was at the centre of progressive thinking. Today, one of the main yardsticks by which a progressive society is measured is the value it places on human life. To give substance to that idea, over many years we have developed institutions and associations dedicated to relieving suffering and saving human life, funded by charity, private enterprise or government.

The first such organisation developed out of efforts to save life at sea on the north-east coast of England. Growth in international trade following the Industrial Revolution led to ever-busier sea ports with an inevitable increase in the number of shipwrecks. The first recorded attempt at providing a rescue service for shipwrecked sailors was in the 1770s in Formby, Lancashire, where a boat was kept on the beach to go to their aid. Shortly afterwards in Bamburgh, Northumberland, a group of public-spirited men, calling themselves the Crew Trust, began patrolling the shore on horseback, acting as lookouts for shipwrecks. This led them to commission a 'lifeboat' – a converted fishing boat with cork gunwales and hollow, watertight compartments at the bow and stern, making it very difficult to turn over and unsinkable, or 'unimmergible' in the words of its designer, a local ship builder, Lionel Lukin.

Lukin's boat was successful and lives were saved, but it was a highly local effort and it took a very visible disaster to raise public consciousness of the true value of lifeboats. In March 1789, the merchant ship *Adventurer* ran aground in a violent storm right in the mouth of the Tyne, just 300 yards from the quayside. As it began to break up, the crew was forced to jump into the sea right in front of a huge crowd which had gathered to watch the spectacle. Local boatmen were encouraged to try and save them, but none would put to sea in such conditions and the crowd simply watched as the men drowned. The perils of the sea were suddenly in the public domain, and the idea of providing lifeboats became very topical.

Having witnessed the tragedy, a group of Newcastle businessmen calling themselves the Gentlemen of the Lawe House got together and funded a competition to design a lifeboat, conceived from scratch and capable of putting to sea in even the foulest weather. There was some controversy about the result of the competition. William Wouldhave, an inventor, based his design on observing the way a ladle used in a public well always floated base down, no matter how it was dropped into the water. It was chosen as the winning design, but the prize of two guineas was halved by the

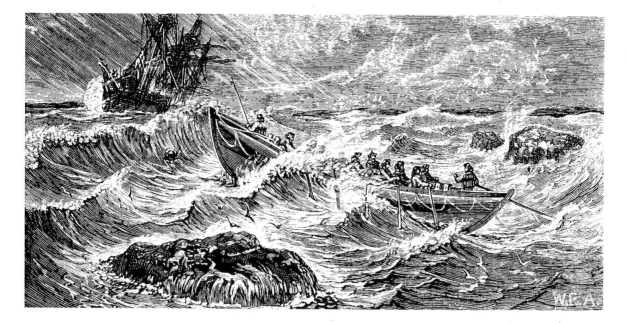

The *Original*, the first true lifeboat, designed by William Wouldhave from scratch to save lives at sea and built by Henry Greathead in Newcastle, going to a stricken ship off the north-east coast of England in 1799.

judges and the contract to build the boat was awarded to Henry Greathead, a boat builder in South Shields. Wouldhave threw the guinea to the floor in disgust on being presented with it.

The *Original*, as the result was christened, was launched in 1790, the first boat in history specifically designed to save lives. It was a thirty-foot rowing boat crewed by ten oarsmen and a coxswain, with seven hundredweight of cork built into it for buoyancy. It could be turned over by very high seas but it would not sink. It saved hundreds of lives off the Tyne estuary over forty years before being wrecked itself. The next step was taken by the Duke of Northumberland who commissioned a second boat from Greathead to be stationed at North Shields where he also left an endowment for its maintenance. In 1800, he paid for a third lifeboat to be stationed in Redcar, where it is still preserved.

The efforts of Tynesiders created an impetus for lifeboats in other parts of the country. Lloyds of London, the marine insurance underwriters, provided £2000 for a further fourteen Greathead lifeboats to be placed at strategic points around the coast, locally manned by volunteer crews. One of the Lloyds-sponsored boats was stationed at Douglas in the Isle of Man, where an eccentric baronet with a taste for adventure, Sir William Hillary, joined the crew. He served with distinction, saving many lives, but he was frustrated by the fragmented organisation of the lifeboat service and saw the problem as the lack of any national body to standardise procedures and to fund development. In 1823, he gathered support from Members of Parliament, the Church and other Establishment figures to launch a nationwide appeal for donations to fund a National Institution for Preservation of Life from Shipwrecks. His appeal was partly based on the economic loss to the nation caused by shipwrecks, but it also stressed the human tragedy of each life lost at sea. The appeal was well supported and a national lifeboat service was founded. The central principles on which it was founded were that it was to be financed by voluntary subscription and the boats were to be manned by volunteers.

Sir William Hillary's creation became the Royal National Lifeboat Institution. High on the list of virtues required to serve in it was physical courage – that quiet courage coupled with modesty and a cool head in a crisis – and to mark that quality in its crews, the RNLI instituted Gold, Silver and Bronze Medals for brave conduct. The first Gold Medal was awarded in 1824 to Captain Charles Freemantle RN who swam to a Swedish brig which had gone aground off Christchurch in Hampshire. He tied a line around his waist and reached the ship in heavy seas as it started to break up. He managed to get the ship's own boats clear but they sank and he found the crew too stunned by the experience to follow his plan to get them ashore, so, unable to do any more, he was hauled back to the beach where he arrived unconscious. The ship did break up and the crew eventually managed to scramble ashore using the fallen mainmast.

In the course of his long career with the RNLI, Sir William

Hillary was involved in rescues which saved 305 people from the sea and he was awarded the Gold Medal three times for rescue work from Douglas and a fourth for founding the Institution.

After the initial period of public enthusiasm, the RNLI went through a period of apathy which lasted into the 1850s, during which it took a subsidy from the government to keep it going. Another disaster which cost the lives of twenty lifeboatmen in the South Shields lifeboat rekindled public support, and ever since the RNLI has been a self-supporting charity. Today there are over 200 lifeboat stations around the coast of the British Isles equipped with powerful motor boats and inshore inflatables to cover holiday beaches. They receive around 5000 calls a year and save some 1500 lives. The tradition of volunteer crews lives on and RNLI lifeboatmen remain some of the most respected members of their

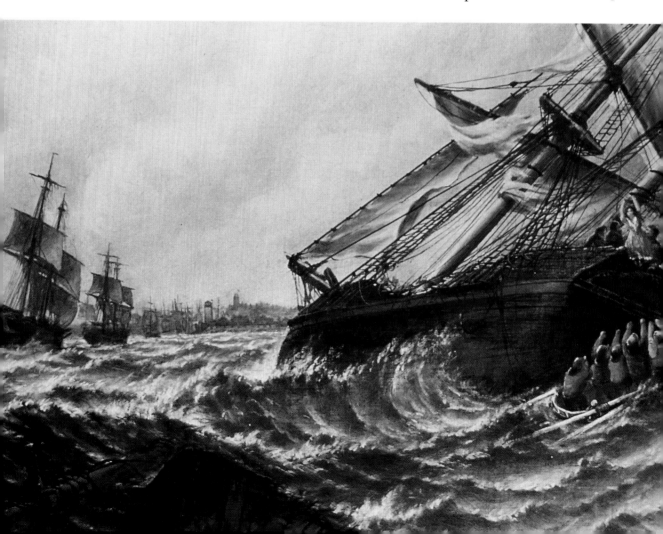

seafaring communities, and indeed throughout the country. The RNLI ethos of volunteering for a dangerous job, and doing so in a spirit of selflessness and professionalism, set many of the standards for making such organisations work and over many years this ethos has spread beyond the lifeboat service to other rescue services as they have evolved.

Alongside the RNLI today is the Coastguard service which was founded in 1820. Its main purpose then was to serve as lookouts for invasion following the Napoleonic wars, but it rapidly adopted a humanitarian role too, monitoring shipping activity for trouble and training in cliff rescue. It has worked closely with the RNLI ever since and is today often first to call out the lifeboats.

During much the same period, another novel and extremely controversial idea began to evolve – the idea of organised civil protection, not from the elements this time, but from crime. As cities expanded during the Industrial Revolution so crime increased in their streets. It was mostly petty crime, but the only response of legislators was to increase the harshness of punishments. By 1799, there were over 200 crimes which carried the death penalty and many more for which people were transported. Law and order had been the responsibility of unpaid parish constables and night watchmen known as 'Charlies', who were incapable of tackling the crime wave. In 1749, the novelist and social reformer, Henry Fielding, who was also a Justice of the Peace in Middlesex and Westminster, established the Bow Street Runners in London. He recruited around 400 men who patrolled the streets under the direction of Middlesex magistrates who were ultimately responsible to the Home Secretary, but neither they nor the 'Charlies' had any statutory powers to stop crime.

There had been a police force in Paris for over a century, but in Britain such a force was seen as having the potential to become an

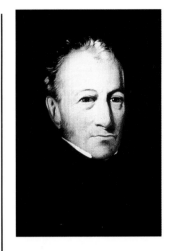

Sir William Hillary, eccentric aristocrat and lifeboat coxswain, who founded the Royal National Lifeboat Institution in 1823.

Opposite page
Lifeboat going to the rescue of a wreck in the mouth of the River Tyne; the provision of lifeboats quickly spread from the North East of England to other parts of the country.

internal army, a way for the government – in the case of France a revolutionary government – to enforce its will on the people. Today we would call such an army a paramilitary force. There was fierce opposition to the idea of forming a similar force in London, even when crime was soaring. Crime was especially prevalent along the Thames waterfront and in 1800 common sense began to prevail with the formation of the first police force in Britain to be given the authority of law – the Marine Police Establishment which came into being under the Thames River Police Act with 60 full-time officers whose duties were to prevent crime in the docks area of London only.

Throughout the 1820s, the momentum behind political and social reform grew, and so did the crime rate. The Home Secretary, Sir Robert Peel, estimated at one point that every twenty-second person in London was involved in crime and that the law-abiding public needed some protection from such an army of criminals. In the teeth of opposition from members of his own Tory party, in particular the hero of Waterloo, the Duke of Wellington, for whom all reform was anathema, Peel eventually secured the agreement of Parliament for an unarmed police force for London.

On 26 September 1829, recruits to the Metropolitan Police, the

'Bobbies', or 'Peelers' as they were popularly known after Sir Robert Peel, the Home Secretary who founded the Metropolitan Police Force in 1829, on parade in regulation top hats.

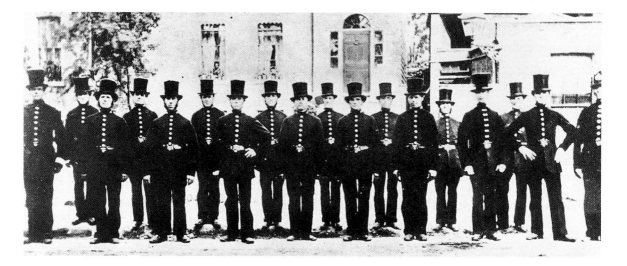

first uniformed, statutory force in Britain, paraded in blue frock coats with numbers embroidered on the lapels outside the Foundling Hospital in Bloomsbury where they took an oath of loyalty. The following Tuesday the first patrols were sent out, starting at 6p.m. Most of the original recruits were discharged for being drunk on duty, but a year later, better recruitment had been established and there were 3250 officers on duty across London, from seventeen district stations, coordinated from a headquarters at 4 Whitehall, next to Great Scotland Yard.

The ethos of a benign force, one which policed with the consent of the public rather than one set in authority over it, was established from the start by the first Commissioners of the Metropolitan Police, Colonel Charles Rowan, another veteran of Waterloo, and a young lawyer, Richard Mayne. Central to their training of policemen was a clear instruction to keep their tempers, to be polite and dignified at all times while cultivating an air of authority backed by law. Once it was clear that the law-abiding public had little to fear from the police and much to gain from their protection, they were accepted, and by 1858, similar though much smaller forces had been established throughout the country.

Today there are 28,000 police officers in the Metropolitan force, on top of a separate, smaller City of London force. Despite years of enormous social and technical change, the essential manner of the British police officer which was established in 1829 remains the same: quiet, assured, polite but firm and, crucially, unarmed. Police forces, backed by most individual police officers, have resisted all attempts in peace time to turn them into a routinely armed force as they understand the value of being unarmed in their relationship with the public. Even today, as police officers increasingly face armed criminals and special units have been formed to carry guns when they are needed, that long tradition seems unlikely to change.

* * *

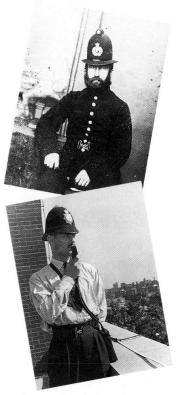

Above: The shape of things to come: in 1864, the Metropolitan police traded in their top hats for the 'coxcomb' helmet.

Below: In 1964, Lancashire police introduced personal radios, a revolution in communications which quickly spread throughout the country, transforming police work.

James Braidwood, the first Superintendent of the London Fire Brigade, who forged a single fire service for the capital out of the many small services. He was also a great innovator, designing breathing apparatus for his men as early as the 1840s.

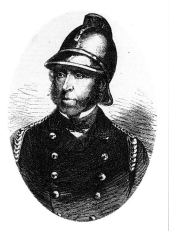

The same tide of reform which created a unified police force brought together the disparate elements which made up London's oldest emergency service, the fire brigades. The first protection against fire had been established in London in 1684, using hand-operated water pumps on wheels manned by part-time and full-time firemen. These 'fire engynes' were maintained by the insurance companies which came into being following the Great Fire of London in 1666. Each company had its men and pumps which only put out fires in buildings bearing the firemark of that insurance company. The idea spread, and by Acts of Parliament in 1707 and 1774 the government ensured that each parish provided its own fire cover with a horse-drawn pump complete with hoses and ladders. The first municipal fire service was set up in Beverley in Yorkshire in 1726, but it took until 1833 for London to get its first citywide fire brigade, the London Fire Engine Establishment. It was formed by merging the insurance companies' individual fire services, which were still paid for by the insurance companies, into a single force with eighty full-time firemen at nineteen stations round the city.

The first Superintendent of the LFEE was James Braidwood, a man of heroic proportions for whom fire fighting was the passion of his life. He was born in Edinburgh where, following the city's own great fire of 1823, he became Superintendent of its fire service at the age of twenty-three. He organised local men into a part-time but trained service, he invented escape ladders and took part in fire fighting himself, on one occasion personally rescuing nine people. He came to London in 1833, the year before the Houses of Parliament were burnt to the ground despite the best efforts of the LFEE firemen. Braidwood warned the Prime Minister, the Duke of Wellington, that London should have its own municipal fire brigade, paid for out of public funds and expanded and organised on a citywide basis like the Metropolitan Police, but his warnings

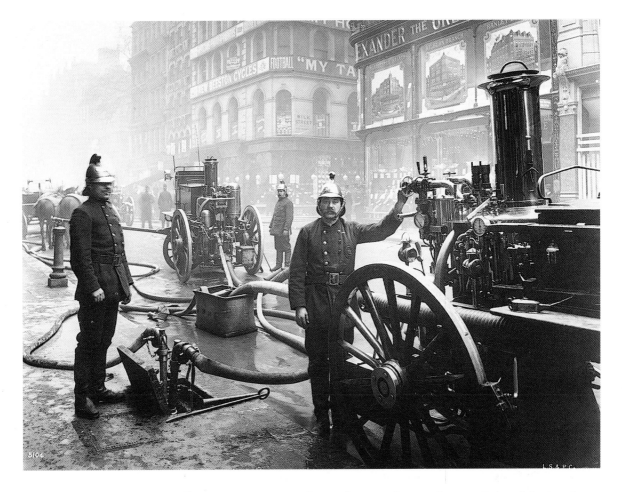

fell on deaf ears. Again Wellington was opposed to reform and saw no reason to change the existing arrangements, despite the huge growth of London and the development of commercial warehouses along the Thames.

It took twenty-eight years and another disaster for the London Fire Brigade to come into existence. On 22 June 1861, a fire started in a riverside warehouse in Tooley Street, just down river from London Bridge. Braidwood could not resist going down to the Thames and directing operations himself and he called out virtually the entire LFEE to fight the fire as it spread along the wharves and warehouses. His efforts were to little avail: as he had warned, the

Members of the London Fire Brigade attending a fire in Bread Street in 1899; horse-drawn fire engines with steam pumps were introduced by James Braidwood in 1861.

35

buildings had grown beyond the range and capacity of his men's equipment and there was just too much combustible material in them. He did his best and was with his firemen going down to the river's edge when a warehouse wall, weakened by the fire, collapsed on top of him and he was killed instantly. His funeral in north London brought out huge crowds and once again made the government think about his ideas for a London Fire Brigade, paid for by the people and the merchants of the city.

The merchants and the insurance companies were by now also behind the idea and urged reform on the government. Following the fire in Tooley Street, insurance premiums rose in leaps and bounds to cover the cost, not only of the fire, but also the cost of improving the fire service. It took another five years for the Metropolitan Fire Brigade to come into being on 1 January 1866.

Gradually, as municipalities grew in importance in the Victorian age, so they organised their own fire services in towns and at their peak there were round 1700 separate services round the country. Some were full time but most were manned by volunteers who had full-time jobs nearby who could get to the fire engine quickly. Technology also improved during Victorian times, steam replacing man power as the source of energy for the pumps. Because these machines were very large and heavy, they were horse drawn, driven at high speed through the streets by teams of specially bred horses. They could be extremely dangerous, occasionally killing firemen who fell off in their high-speed dashes to fires. For their heroic image and endeavours, the men of the Metropolitan Fire Brigade became real heroes to the population of London.

Braidwood was succeeded as London's Chief Fire Officer by Captain Eyre Massey Shaw, a man equally absorbed by the art of fire fighting. He too was innovative and led from the front, directing the fire engines as well as looking after his office duties. At the height of Victorian England in the 1870s his big, burly firemen,

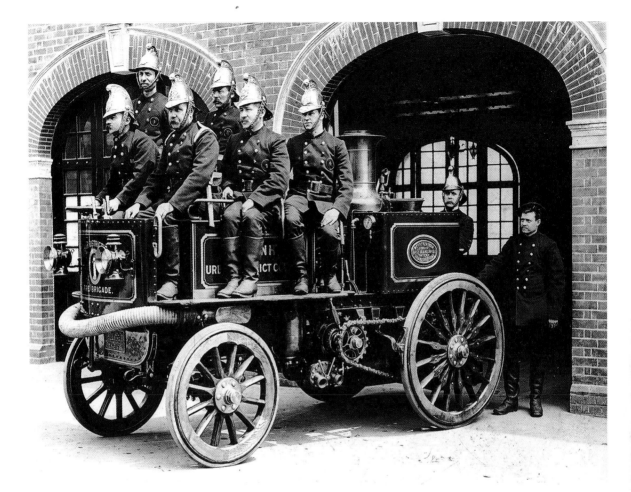

dressed in their blue uniforms with long boots and topped with magnificent, heavily decorated, gleaming brass helmets reminiscent of Norse gods, charging noisily through the streets on their way to a fire became one of the sights of London. Shaw also cultivated Royal patronage and the Prince of Wales, later Edward VII, took a keen interest in their work and was not above going to a fire in full regalia, giving the fire service a status and an esprit de corps to match that of the finest regiments in the British Army. On the day of his retirement, 30 October 1891, Captain Shaw was knighted by Queen Victoria.

* * *

A self-propelled Merryweather fire engine of 1903; Merryweather have been builders of fire fighting equipment since 1692.

Of all the emergency services, the ambulance service is the most obviously humanitarian, but the idea of vehicles to carry patients to hospital, either from their homes or from the scene of an accident, took a long time to evolve in Britain. Once again the original idea came from France. The first ambulances were designed for Napoleon's army – horse-drawn carriages with highly sprung boxes on top to carry wounded soldiers from the battlefield to hospital. They were designed by Napoleon's personal doctor, Dominique Jean Larrey, and organised into an ambulance corps by the Chief Surgeon of the French Army in 1796. Napoleon's great opponent and an opponent of most reform, the Duke of Wellington, refused to have an organised ambulance corps in the British Army.

It was not until the Crimean War in 1854, two years after the Duke's death, that the Hospital Conveyance Corps, employing Army pensioners, was organised to help British soldiers. The appalling suffering and the neglect which soldiers endured, from wounds or more often through disease, horrified humanitarians. One of their number, Florence Nightingale, overturned the reactionary ideas of senior soldiers and many Army doctors by cleaning up the hospital at Scutari in the Crimea and providing nursing care. Florence Nightingale was one of the early proponents of humanitarian ideals, in peace as well as in war, at a time when the idea of relieving human suffering was growing throughout Europe.

The movement culminated in 1864 when the nations gathered in Geneva to sign an international convention regulating the treatment of prisoners of war and the treatment of civilians in war time. It was in response to the horrors of the Crimean War and in particular those of the United States Civil War, in which the battles and the suffering of the soldiers had been widely photographed, increasing public awareness of exactly what went on in war. The Geneva Convention was a landmark in the consolidation of humanitarian ideas, but to give the theory a practical means of relieving suffering, the Red Cross was formed in the same year by a Swiss humanitarian Jean Henri Dunant, who had organised aid for both French and Austrian soldiers at the Battle of Solferino that year. The Red Cross symbol, a symmetrical red cross on a white background, is the reverse of the Swiss flag and has ever since been used to identify ambulances, hospitals and other non-combatant installations.

The foundation of the Red Cross triggered a burgeoning of humanitarian organisations in Europe. In Britain, one man became the driving force behind the creation of a practical answer to humanitarian problems. John Furley, who was born in 1836 and spent much of his early adult life as a soldier, had seen both the suffering of soldiers and the impact of war on civilian populations caught up in it. In the same year that the Geneva Convention was signed, he joined the Order of St John, an ancient, Christian order of chivalry dedicated to relieve suffering by building hospitals. In 1869 he pledged the Order to founding a National Aid Society, and he was instrumental in founding the British Red Cross in 1870 and the British National Association for Aid to the Sick and Wounded – all of them funded by charitable donation and relying on volunteers. He was, like Braidwood of the fire service, also an inventor of devices to aid suffering: an 'ambulance hamper', or what we would call a first aid kit; a portable electric light for searching battlefields for wounded; a single-wheeled litter for transporting patients.

In 1877, Furley committed the Order to being the instrument through which Britain would have a nationwide ambulance service. The Ambulance Association was formed that year under the auspices of the Order of St John, principally to provide people trained in emergency medical treatment or, as it quickly became known, first aid. The idea was to train people in simple medical attention which could stabilise an injured person or in extreme cases preserve

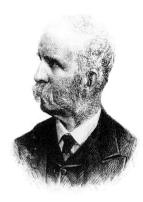

Sir John Furley, a former soldier turned humanitarian, was a member of the Order of St John and the Red Cross. He led the foundation of ambulance services in Britain, combining great organisational skill with technical innovation.

their life before taking them to hospital for professional treatment. The first classes for teaching first aid were held by the Surgeon-Major Peter Shepherd of the Ambulance Association in Woolwich. In 1878, he published the first textbook on first aid under the title *Aids for Cases of Injuries and Sudden Illness* to spread the word.

The following year, the first ambulance station was established by the Association at Margate in Kent. The man behind that was a local bookseller, William Church Brazier, a man dedicated to the idea of voluntary service; he was a local part-time fireman and worked closely with the Margate lifeboat. His first ambulance was one of John Furley's single-wheeled litters but by 1883 Furley had designed a well-sprung horse-drawn ambulance with rubber tyres which could carry four stretchers and first-aid-trained attendants to look after the patients in transit.

The next stage was to spread the work throughout the country and this the Order did by establishing local branches, especially in the north of England among the industrial working classes who

John Furley designed the first British ambulance for the Invalid Transport Corps which he formed in 1883 to provide transport to hospital for the poor. The well-sprung, horse-drawn carriage was built of ash, with a mahogany finish inside with room for three patients on stretchers and a single first-aid attendant.

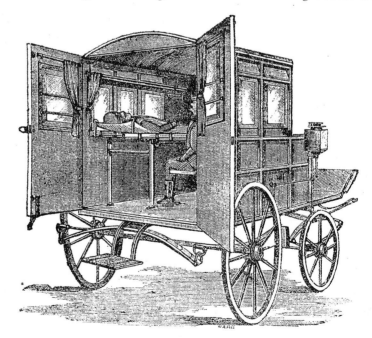

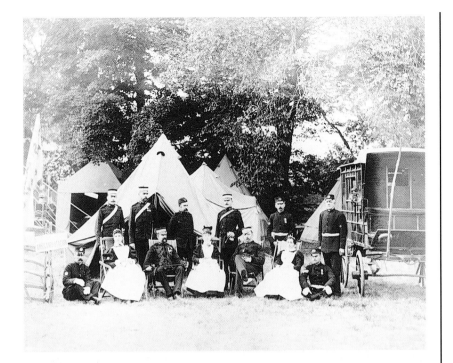

St John Ambulance Station: William Church Brazier (fourth from left, standing) who founded the first organised ambulance service in Margate, Kent in 1879, with his team of first aiders and nurses.

supported the ambulance movement and benefited from it. In 1885, there were over 8000 industrial accidents in Britain resulting in 407 fatalities. The St John Ambulance Brigade provided not only first-aid training which was of great value in the workplace and ambulances to take injured people to hospital, it also moved into the provision of medical aids such as crutches and Bath chairs for the poor. In 1866, the Order founded the Invalid Transport Corps to provide a national body for ambulance work and by 1888 there were 100,000 volunteers nationwide. John Furley's energy and organisational ability provided the country with a voluntary ambulance service which was quickly absorbed into British life.

In the 1890s, a revolution began in transport which was eventually to have far-reaching effects on all the emergency services. The internal combustion engine began to replace the horse, providing

Emergency ambulance service 1884: an unsprung litter pushed by a policeman through the streets of Manchester from the scene of a rail crash to the Royal Infirmary.

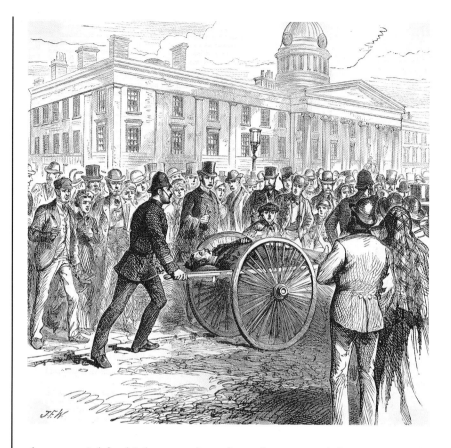

the potential for higher speeds and much more mobility in responding to emergencies. The first prototype motor ambulance was exhibited in Paris in 1895 and the first self-propelled fire engine in 1898. The first recorded use of the police using a car to chase and catch a criminal was in 1899 in Northampton; Sergeant McLeod borrowed a Benz belonging to a local businessman, Jack Harrison, and chased a man who had been selling forged tickets for Barnum & Bailey's circus. The speed limit at the time was 12mph and it was probably broken in the chase, but the fugitive was arrested.

France was the first country to adopt motorised ambulances both for military and civilian use, the earliest type coming into service in 1900. It was a motor-driven tractor which carried a doctor and a driver, with the patient in a box on wheels towed behind it. Britain followed in 1905 when the Metropolitan Asylums Board in London bought a motor ambulance to carry scarlet fever patients from their homes to isolation hospitals in south London. In 1907, the City of London Police introduced a motorised ambulance service using electric vehicles. They did so in conjunction with another technological advance, the telephone, by establishing a network of fifty-two emergency telephone boxes across the city from which people could call for assistance. Motorised ambulances made great advances during the First World War in which many of the St John volunteers served. In 1919, the Ambulance Association formed the Home Ambulance Service with 264 motor ambulances nationwide used mainly to carry the sick to and from hospital. It was the forerunner of the modern service.

The first motorised fire engine in Britain was a Daimler which carried six men of the Liverpool Fire Brigade in 1901. It backfired frequently and was known as 'Farting Annie' and was used for the first time to go to a fire in a cotton warehouse; the horse-drawn engine from the same fire station got to the fire first. Speed was of the essence in getting to a fire and as petrol-driven fire engines improved in speed and reliability so they steadily replaced the horse in the first two decades of the new century, the last horse-drawn machine being pensioned off in 1921. The new machines, generally painted red with gleaming lights and polished brass, on which the firemen sat in the race to a fire, lost none of the appeal of the horse-drawn era and the firemen lost nothing of their heroic image.

The main task of firemen has always been and still is to fight fires, but because of the public-spirited men the service attracted and because of the equipment they carried on the tenders, firemen also became rescuers of people from all kinds of accidents and perilous circumstances. For example, as cities built sewers to improve public health, one of the fire brigade's many tasks was to rescue sewer workers who had been overcome by fumes. A tragic incident occurred in March 1913 when a sewer worker was overcome in Bayswater and firemen from Notting Hill went to the scene at Pembridge Villas. They had just been issued with oxygen breathing apparatus for the purpose and two of them, Fireman Libby and Fireman McLaren, went down and found the man, William Parry. They tried to revive him by removing one of their masks and forcing it into his mouth but in the process both the firemen were overcome by the fumes and collapsed. More firemen went down to rescue them and brought all three men out, but they were dead.

Fire services developed specialised rescue tenders for such work which carried all sorts of other equipment, from portable floodlights to hydraulic jacks and cutting equipment, breathing apparatus and folding canvas stretchers to get injured people out of restricted areas. Rescue rather than fire was the reason for the London Fire Brigade being called to an incident in Kilburn in October 1923, where a five-storey building collapsed while builders were working inside it, trapping fifteen men. Firemen were on the spot very quickly and they were confronted by a mass of tangled steel scaffolding and brickwork. Removing people from a collapsed building is very intricate work; moving any piece of the tangle may disturb the whole structure and bring more down on the heads of the trapped men. It took hours to work their way through it safely, but all the men survived.

The first police cars were twelve Fords bought in 1919 to transport senior officers rather than chase criminals. The first mobile police unit was formed by the CID in 1920, twelve detectives using ex-RAF Crossley vans. Each vehicle was equipped with a radio, another new technology which would grow in importance to the emergency services. They were used as covert observation posts, disguised as milk floats or delivery vans, but the huge, square aerials on their roofs gave them away and professional criminals

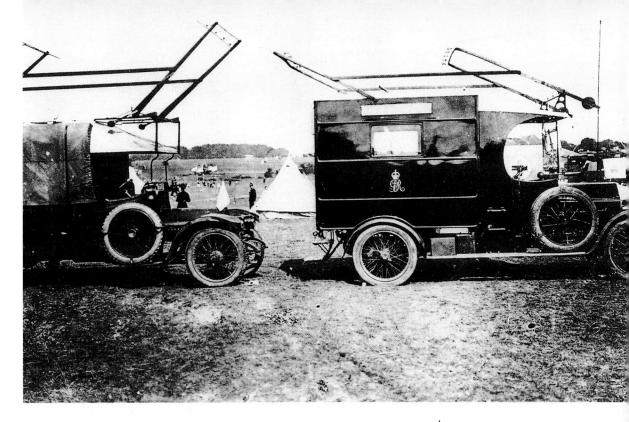

christened them 'Flying Bedsteads'. The press christened the unit the 'Flying Squad' or even more famously the 'Sweeney' as it quickly became known in East London.

By 1930 police cars were in regular use for patrolling and in the same year the Metropolitan Police introduced motorcycles as well. Two years later, police cars equipped with radios were introduced in Lancashire and in 1934 the Metropolitan Police introduced the first twenty-four-hour patrols by radio-equipped cars, one car to each of fifty-two designated areas.

The idea of vehicles equipped with radio was the start of a mobility and communications revolution for the emergency services. On 1 July 1937 came a landmark in the development of an organised response to emergencies, the first emergency telephone. By dialling 999 members of the public could be put through instantly to the police, fire or ambulance services and the system remains today as the main link between people in distress and the rescue services.

The first radio-equipped police vehicles at Epsom for Derby Day in 1923; they were ex-RAF Crossley tenders known as Flying Bedsteads from the huge wireless aerials on the roof.

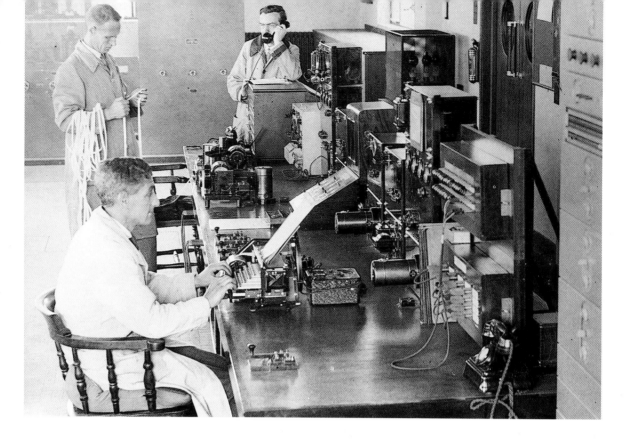

Communications revolution: one of the first police control rooms at West Wickam, Kent, first used in 1937.

During the Second World War, all three 999 services were in the front line on the home front. The humanitarian response to war, especially to the reality of large-scale aerial bombing of civilian targets, transformed the fire service in particular. The last insurance company fire brigade had only been disbanded in 1929 by Norwich Union in Worcester, but there were still some 1650 individual services around the country, each with its own way of doing things. None of them would be able to cope with a major emergency and would rely on neighbouring services which operated using different drill with different equipment. War galvanised thinking, and the need for standardisation and massive expansion became the priority. During the Blitz of 1940–41, the hundreds of fire brigades were nationalised, becoming the National Fire Service on 18 August 1940. In addition to the 118,000 full-time firemen, 240,000 part-time fire fighters were recruited into the Auxiliary Fire Service, including 60,000 women.

War had come to the home front, and to recognise civilian acts of conspicuous bravery in the same way that the Victoria Cross did for military and naval action, the George Cross was introduced on 23 September 1940. Only a few days before it was instituted, there was an example of the reason why it should exist. During an air raid on the night of 17–18 September, a number of auxiliary firemen were sheltering in the basement of a garage being used as a temporary fire station. Around midnight, the building took a direct hit, killing twenty people. Fireman Harry Errington was knocked unconscious and when he came to the building was on fire. Nearby was a colleague trapped by fallen debris and another under a radiator. He carried them to safety one at a time up a narrow staircase at the back of the building. All three men were badly burned and had to go to hospital but made complete recoveries. Harry Errington was awarded the George Cross, but after a statutory period of thirteen weeks to recover, he was also discharged from the service as a result of his injuries.

Another George Cross was awarded to Anthony Smith, a chimney sweep serving with the Heavy Rescue Squad which was formed to extricate people from bombed buildings. On 23 February 1944, a block of flats was hit in Chelsea and escaping gas set the remains of the building alight. Smith dug his way into a front basement to rescue a trapped man. With fire all around him and walls falling in from above, he brought the man out, then went back into the building with a colleague and spent over an hour extricating another victim.

There were many acts of bravery during the War, and the spirit of a single, dedicated service became embedded in the Fire Service, as did the front-line mentality. At a house fire in Shepherd's Bush on 22 August 1945, which was so fierce it seemed impossible for anybody to enter the building, fireman Frederick Davies climbed a ladder and went into a bedroom, returning moments later with a

Overleaf: Some of the 20,000 firemen in the City of London during one of the heaviest raids of the Blitz on 29–30 December 1940. The raid was timed to coincide with the low tide of the Thames, bombs then smashed the water mains before 10,000 incendiary bombs set the city alight, forcing the firemen to wade into the Thames mud to pump water.

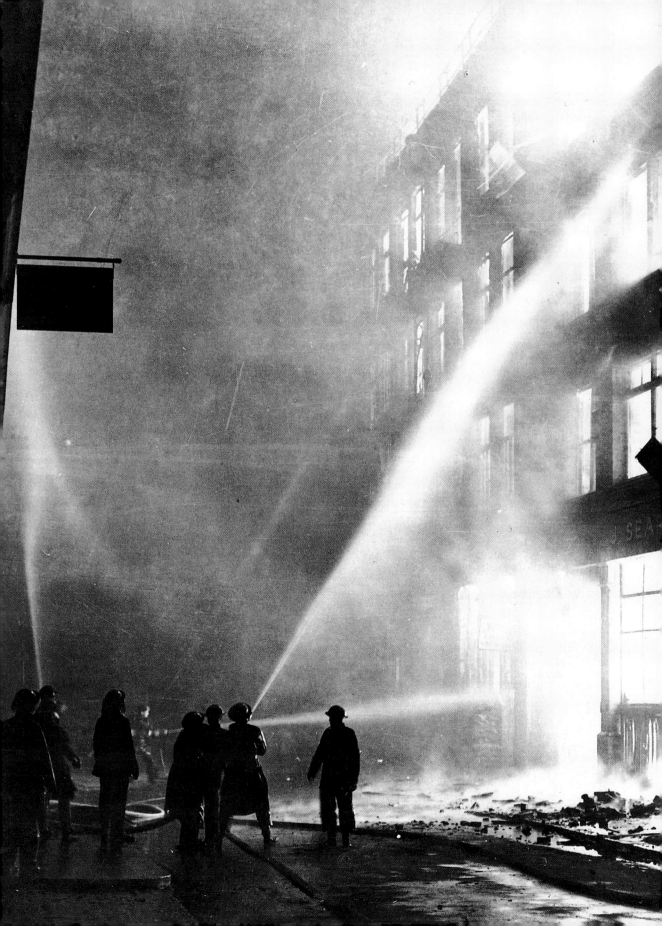

child which he handed to a colleague. He was ordered out, but re-entered the building bringing out a second child who was dead. His clothes were on fire from head to foot and he was rushed to hospital where he died from his injuries. He was awarded the George Cross posthumously.

The post-war Labour government reformed many aspects of life in Britain and the emergency services were no exception. It took the idea of a National Fire Service and retained the common standards of training and equipment, but divided it up between the local authorities by Act of Parliament in 1947. Many of the firemen were full time but the spirit of the professional volunteer, which had been the backbone of the service for over a century, lived on, particularly in rural areas where the service was based on 'retained' or part-time firemen who worked near their stations and would leave their jobs and rush to man the engines when they heard the siren.

One of the post-war Labour government's greatest reforms was the creation of the Welfare State and with it the National Health Service. Despite opposition from the medical profession, Britain's 2751 hospitals were nationalised in 1948 and day-to-day running

Below: Home Front: London's rescue services faced a huge new task in July 1944 when a second Blitz, this time from flying bombs launched in France, destroyed over 200,000 houses and killed 1,700 people in two weeks. The government decided to evacuate mothers and children under five and one million people had been moved to the country before the raids stopped.

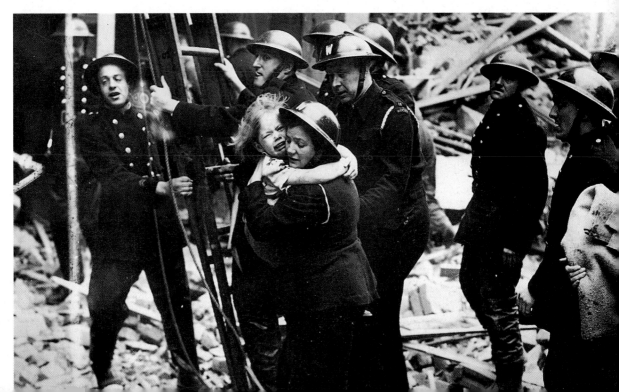

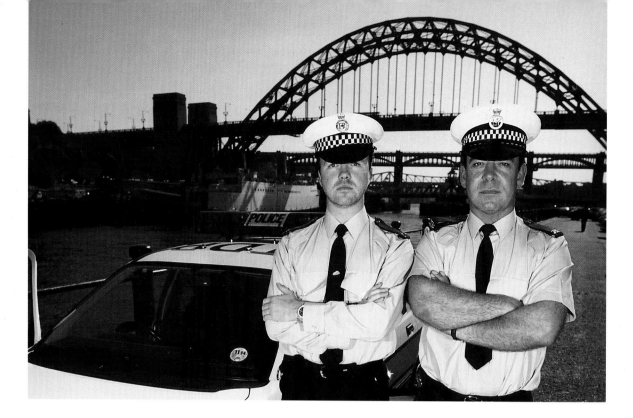

PC Simon Pawsey (left) and his partner PC Brian English, traffic policemen with the Northumbria Police, featured in a dramatic car chase in their Ford Sierra Cosworth to arrest drug dealers being followed by undercover police in the first series of *Blues and Twos*. Following that incident, they were called to a hospital where a man was threatening to hang himself; they talked him out of it.

of health services was put under the control of local Health Authorities, paid for by public funds rather than charity. At the same time, the new bodies took over the provision of ambulance services from the St John Ambulance Brigade, in some cases literally taking over established St John vehicles and premises.

As the post-war world became more and more complex so the evolution of the emergency services has been driven by two factors: greater use of technology and higher levels of professional training. In the 1950s, for example, at a major train crash, members of the public would be on the scene in large numbers helping to clear debris and care for the injured. Today, an incident however large or small is cordoned off, the province of the emergency services only.

The three 999 services work closely together, especially in major incidents. A major road traffic accident, especially a multiple pile-up on a motorway, will certainly involve all three, each with their own areas of expertise: the police have the authority to control the situation, divert traffic, keep crowds away, and look for evidence if the incident has legal implications; ambulance staff and paramedics provide emergency medical aid and evacuate the injured; and firemen, once any fire hazard is under control, become the general practitioners of the rescue business, ready for anything. Most fire fighters are fit, tough men and women with a keenness to get on with the job, always able to find the right piece of equipment or improvise if necessary. The fire services' rescue tenders have become mobile rescue workshops with electrical, hydraulic and air lines to operate halogen floodlights, spreading and cutting equipment, air bags to open out crashed vehicles to release injured people, power tools and lifting gear. Motorway crashes can hold lethal surprises. As the chemical industry carries more and more of

From the first series of *Blues and Twos*: paramedic Derek Young and ambulance technician Steve Watkins of the Edinburgh Ambulance Service, one of the busiest ambulance services in the country. Steve has since retrained as a paramedic and will feature in the second series.

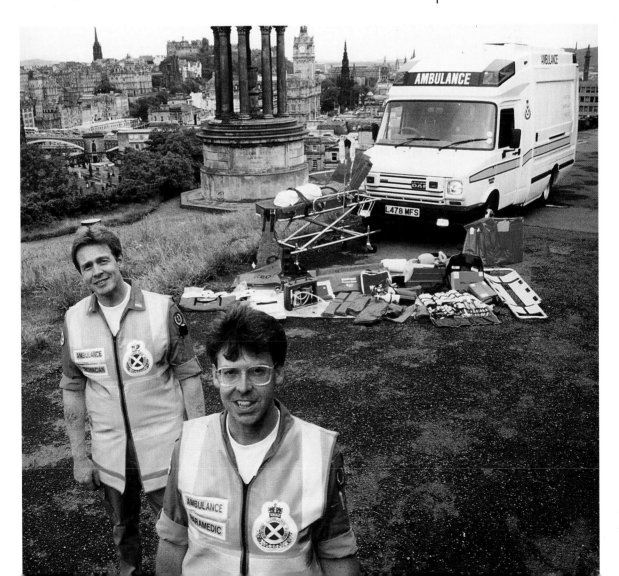

its products by road, when their trucks crash there is not only greater danger of fire, there could also be toxic substances and somebody has to deal with them. From the 1960s, fire brigades have carried equipment to check for radiation, and suits incorporating breathing apparatus to encase the wearer completely have enabled firemen to continue to deal with even the most hazardous situations.

Mobility and communications have continued to improve and they have become the basis of much emergency work. In 1965, the Lancashire police introduced the first panda cars, giving virtually every police officer access to mobility. At the same time, personal radios were introduced. Today strapping on a radio and going on the beat with an earpiece tuned permanently to the local police network is as routine as putting on the uniform.

Ambulances carry ever more life-saving equipment and ambulance crews are able to provide much more than first aid; in some cases paramedics carry out what amounts to surgery on the pavement. Of today's nearly 11,000 front-line ambulance officers approximately half are paramedics and the target is for 60 per cent by the end of 1995. In major emergencies, they are backed up by doctors trained in emergency procedures with experience of working in disasters, belonging to an organisation called BASICS, the British Association for Immediate Care.

After sixty years, even the 999 service is changing. Instead of being simply a means of contact between the public and the emergency services, it is beginning to provide emergency medical advice over the phone. Using a system called Emergency Medical Despatch, which originated in America and was pioneered in this country by the Derbyshire Ambulance Service, the 999 operator no longer simply takes the message and sends an ambulance to the address. Now they stay on the line, asking questions about the casualty, reassuring the caller and giving specific medical advice from a computer database even before the ambulance arrives.

Above all else, the emergency services have grown. Taken together their strength represents around 75 per cent of the total size of Britain's armed forces. In 1995, the thirty-seven ambulance services in England employ 17,850 people making 17 million patient journeys a year, 2 million of them as a result of 999 calls. The fire service in England and Wales employs 34,700 full-time fire fighters and 15,054 part-time 'retained' firemen backed up by 1545 control staff. The police force employs 125,350 full-time police officers backed up by 13,340 special constables and 46,181 civilian staff. In addition to the three 999 services the RNLI, Coastguard, Air/Sea Rescue services of the RAF and Royal Navy, mountain rescue teams and cave rescue bring the total to around 300,000. The costs have also risen. Emergency work is expensive: the budget for the ambulance service in England is £508m and its 999 service consumes 80 per cent of it; the fire service costs £1.61bn a year; the police £6.5bn.

Rescue and civil protection are integral parts of a modern society, an industry, almost, in its own right. They are constantly seeking to use new technologies to improve and expand the range of what they do. Behind the front-line staff is a huge infrastructure of specialist suppliers, staff colleges for senior officers, training courses, trade unions, press officers, trade magazines with annual conferences, international conventions and seminars. Britain is a world leader in rescue techniques and equipment, but few who know the services would disagree that this position has been built on the tradition of selflessness, voluntary spirit and a willingness to face disaster which has always been at the heart of our emergency services.

In a world where popular culture has replaced values of service and selflessness and the move to full-time, professional services has changed many aspects of their recruitment, training and experience, the origins of the modern services in the age of Enlightenment, in the humanitarian movement and in the wartime spirit of public service and pulling together are still evident in the people. The men and women in any police, ambulance or fire service tea room today would not have been out of place in any part of their history.

Chapter Three

INDUSTRIAL DISEASE

One of the enduring themes in the development of the modern world has been the quest for new and cheaper sources of energy. Advanced economies such as Britain's have been built on continuous and reliable supplies first of coal, then oil and gas and more recently nuclear power, used to generate electricity. Providing that power is dangerous work and as is so often the case, improvements in safety only come in the wake of disasters and the loss of many lives.

Mining coal has employed millions of miners over the last two centuries, people working thousands of feet underground surrounded by danger from falls of rock and coal, collapsing roofs, fires and gas explosions. Even in countries where safety precautions are generally good, many thousands of miners have died. In this century on 22 December 1910, 350 men died in an explosion at West Houghton mine, near Bolton, leaving over 1000 children orphaned. On 14 October 1913, 418 died at Sengenhydd mine in South Wales in an explosion which was heard 11 miles away in Cardiff. In 1934, 262 men died at Gresford colliery, Wrexham in a fire. Since the Second World War, 80 miners were killed in an explosion underground at Cresswell colliery in Derbyshire in 1950

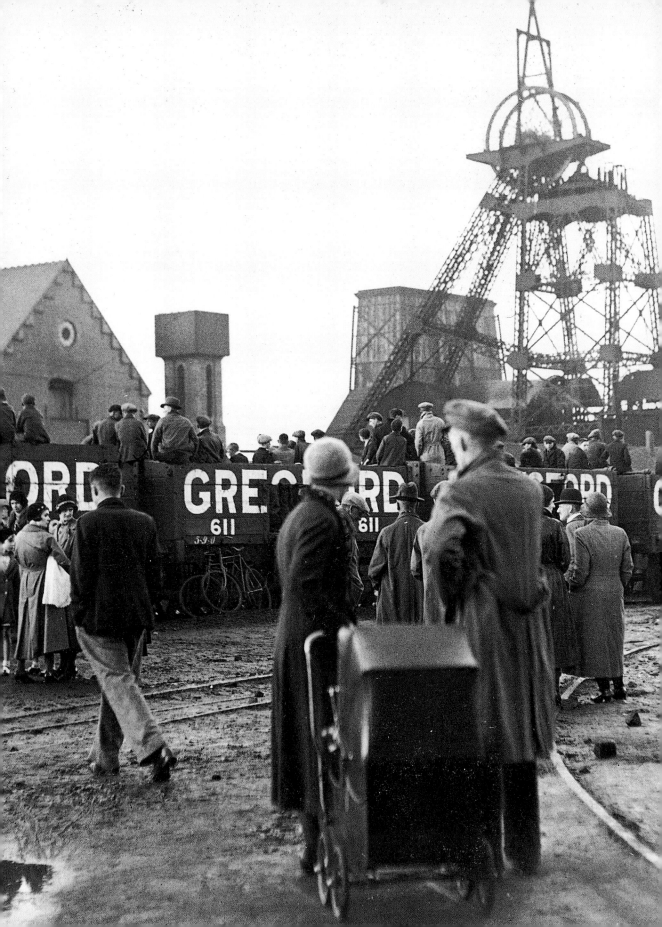

and the following year 83 died at Easington in County Durham, then in June 1960, 28 died at Six Bells colliery in Monmouthshire.

Rescuing trapped miners is a specialised task carried out by teams drawn from the ranks of miners themselves, men who are expert in their jobs. Such teams have saved many lives, though there is little anybody can do in a large explosion. When disasters strike mining communities, they are devastating because all the men live and work together, then they die together, leaving their families to grieve together. Mining families live with disasters, but nothing could have prepared the people of a small mining village in South Wales for what happened on Friday 21 October 1966.

It was the last morning of school before half term at Pantglas Junior School in Aberfan, a large mining village between Merthyr and Pontypridd. The village was wet; it had been raining hard for several days. Above and behind the school towered the giant tips of refuse from the coal mine which had been piling up for over seventy years. School started at 9a.m. There were 199 children on the register and teachers were calling out names at 9.15 when a forty-foot-high section of the coal waste, some two million tons of wet, black slurry, started sliding downhill towards the village half a mile away. On its way down the slope it engulfed a farm, smashed a water main, then hit the school and the surrounding cottages. A great rattling, swishing sound could be heard as the landslide smashed windows and poured into buildings, covering a row of cottages in Moy Road, then a row of shops. Water from the broken main poured down the mountain turning the mixture into the consistency of wet cement. It engulfed the school, then started creeping up and around it, trapping the children and teachers. The secondary school nearby was untouched and the five–seven-year-olds at Pantglas did not start school until later in the morning, so they escaped. Some children were able to climb out of the windows and three classes, totalling 88 children, came out in comparative safety.

Opposite: Pithead vigil: families and colleagues wait for news during a fire at the Gresford Colliery in Wrexham in 1934 in which 262 men died.

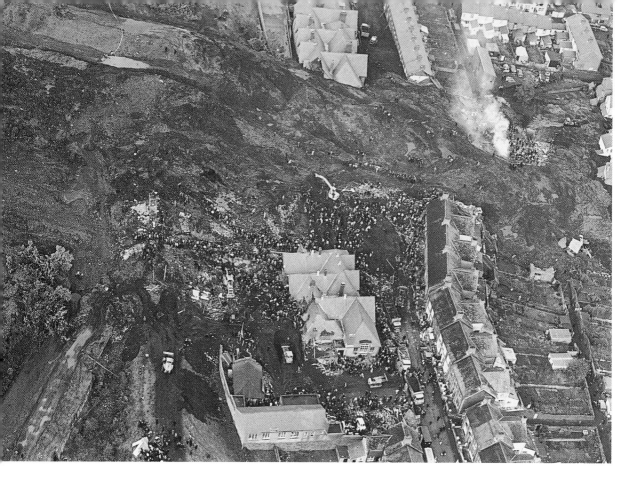

Miners, rescue workers and local volunteers with earth-moving equipment, swarm round Pantglas school in Aberfan in a desperate attempt to rescue children trapped in their classrooms by a tide of coal waste which hit the village on 21 October 1966.

Mrs Emily Griffiths of Pantglas Road dialled 999 and Mrs Gwyneth Davies rang all the emergency services, but it was local people who were first on the scene. A teacher from the secondary school saw five boys swamped by the slurry and he could hear them screaming underneath it. He rushed forward with a colleague into the sludge to try and help but could do nothing. Inside the school, a teacher told her children to crouch on the floor as the classroom began to collapse around them, then she smashed a window and passed some of them to a caretaker outside. An elderly bus conductor who lived in Moy Road heard children screaming and rushed into the street to see the black tide creeping round the school. He ran to it, smashed a window with a chair, crawled in and brought out six children. Mothers with children at Pantglas School rushed to the scene and started digging with their bare

one, responding purposefully to a new and murderous dimension to their work, one for which they would have to constantly learn new skills and face new dangers.

On 26 February 1975, twenty-one-year-old PC Stephen Tibble was off duty and riding his motor bike in Charleville Road, Hammersmith, when he saw a group of colleagues chasing a man along the road. He overtook them on his bike, parked further up the road, then turned to face the fugitive, an IRA suspect, who drew a gun and shot the young policeman twice at point-blank range. PC Tibble died in Charing Cross Hospital later the same day.

On 28 August 1975, a warning was sent to the Metropolitan Police concerning a suspicious package left in a shop doorway in Kensington. Police officers inspected it and saw a watch taped to the top. They closed off the immediate area and called for police bomb disposal officer Roger Goad. The area was evacuated before he started work, but when he bent over to start defusing it, the package exploded and he was killed instantly. Roger Goad was posthumously awarded the George Cross.

On Saturday 7 December, four men in a stolen Ford Cortina drove past Scott's Restaurant in Mayfair and raked it with gunfire, then sped off. A description of the men was quickly sent over the police radio network and two unarmed officers on foot patrol spotted the car in Portman Square. They followed it in a taxi into the Marylebone area. The men in the car fired at them, then abandoned the car as two vans carrying officers of the Special Patrol Group arrived. Shots were exchanged as the men raced into the basement of a block of council flats in Balcombe Street. There was no way out, so they burst into a first-floor flat where they took Mr John Matthews, a Post Office manager, and his wife Sheila, hostage. The police knew they were armed and believed they were IRA terrorists so they surrounded the block, emptied the adjoining flats, closed off all the surrounding streets and settled down for a siege.

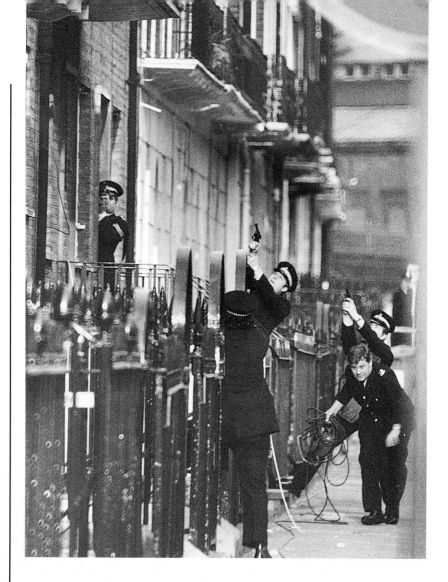

Balcombe Street, London, 8 December 1975: armed police take aim at the window of the flat where four IRA gunmen were holding a couple hostage as a colleague moves up with equipment.

Inside the flat the IRA men barricaded themselves and their two hostages in the sitting room which measured twelve feet by fourteen feet; six people and no lavatory. The first contact was by telephone when a police officer dialled the Matthews' number and spoke to Mr Matthews. The police quickly arranged for the line to be cut off and replaced it with another under their control, lowering the receiver on to the Matthews' balcony from the flat above. Over the phone, the terrorists demanded a car to take them to an aircraft to fly them to the Irish Republic. The police made it plain from the start that no deal would be offered. They also denied the terrorists food, sending in only small amounts of drinking water and a chemical lavatory.

The police technique was to settle down for a long haul: they started fortifying the area around the flat with sandbag emplacements at strategic points manned by armed police officers from D.11, the Metropolitan Police firearms unit. What amounted to a small, sandbagged fort was built right outside the flat on the landing, facing the door. Other specialist police units started to insert tiny listening devices and television cameras through parts of the building to watch and listen to the terrorists' plans, to judge their

Balcombe Street, 12 December 1975: the moment of surrender as one of the terrorists puts his hands over his head while covered by a police marksman.

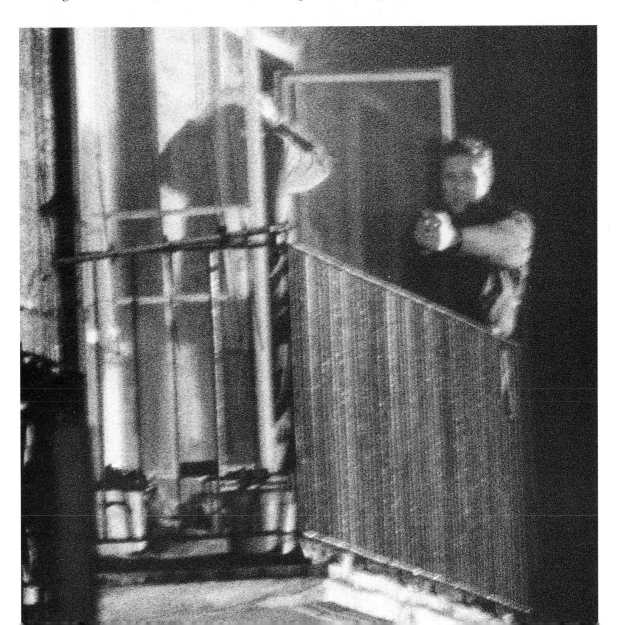

mood, and to decide how best to apply psychological pressure. A unit of the Army's Special Air Service (the SAS) was put on standby, but the operation remained under the control of the police. The siege grew in size: control vans and a mobile canteen drew up and parked in neighbouring streets followed by television trucks parked behind the police cordon, with journalists and press photographers.

The first crack in the terrorists' resolve came after six days when the police offered to swap a hot meal for Mrs Matthews. They agreed, and two and a half hours later a surrender was agreed over the telephone and they came out one by one on to the balcony and were handcuffed to spontaneous cheers from the street below. Forensic evidence linked the men and their weapons to other terrorist acts, including the assassination of Ross MacWhirter, an outspoken journalist, and they were sentenced to life imprisonment with a recommendation that they serve no fewer than thirty years.

On 26 October 1981, the IRA planted three bombs in shops in the West End of London, but there was no specific warning as to where they were so the police had to search for them. A policeman found one in a lavatory in a Wimpy Bar in Oxford Street. The building was quickly evacuated and a Metropolitan Police bomb expert, Kenneth Howorth, went in to investigate. The bomb exploded and killed him instantly. A colleague, Peter Gurney, went to Debenhams department store to deal with a similar device knowing that Mr Howorth was dead. He defused it. Kenneth Howorth was awarded the George Cross posthumously and Peter Gurney, who had already won the George Medal and the MBE for his work in Northern Ireland, was awarded a bar to his George Medal.

The penultimate Saturday before Christmas 1983 was 17 December and Harrods department store in Knightsbridge was packed with 10,000 shoppers. At 12.44p.m., the IRA made a telephone call to the Samaritans, using a designated code word to identify it as a genuine IRA warning. They announced that there were bombs both inside and outside Harrods and in Oxford Street, London's busiest shopping area. The Samaritans called Scotland Yard which immediately put the Anti-Terrorist Squad and Chelsea police station on alert. Chelsea in turn passed the warning on to Harrods staff and at 1.05, a coded message was sent out over the store's public address system, alerting all senior managers to search for bombs. The staff discreetly searched the building, looking in lavatories, pianos and behind serving counters, but they found nothing. As police officers were converging on Knightsbridge, one strong instinct would have been to make an announcement and clear the store, but experience had shown that creating such panic was probably just what the IRA wanted, flooding the streets outside with people, right into the path of a car bomb.

At 1.20, a police car from Chelsea police station with an inspector, a dog handler, a sergeant and a WPC pulled up in Hans

Knightsbridge, 17 December 1983: a photograph taken seconds after the explosion which killed five people, three of them police officers.

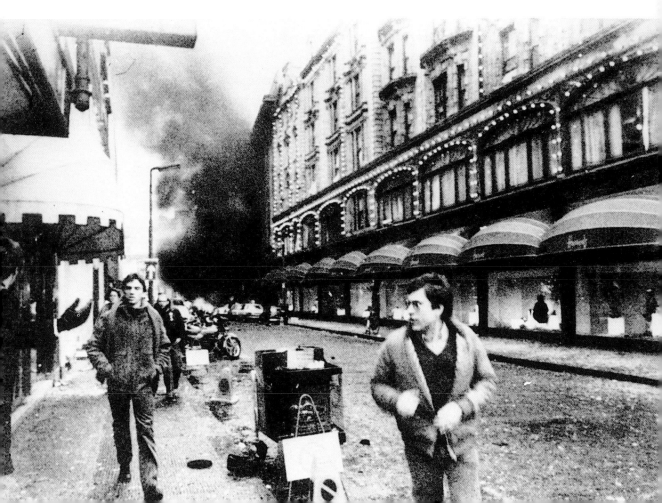

Crescent to one side of the Harrods building. They double-parked beside a blue Austin 1300 and just as they got out of the car, the Austin exploded. Sergeant Noel Land was killed instantly; WPC Jane Arbuthnot was hurled across the street where she died later; and Inspector Stephen Dodd was severely injured – he died later in hospital. Others in the immediate vicinity of the bomb were hurled around like rag dolls. The huge glass windows of Harrods crashed into the street. Ambulances were on the scene quickly and started ferrying the injured to St Thomas's, St Stephen's and Westminster hospitals. Five people died, including the police officers, and ninety-one were injured, among them thirteen more police officers, four of them seriously. Had the store been emptying of people, the death toll would have been far higher.

Nearly a year later, the IRA made a supreme effort to intimidate the British government into changing its policy on Northern Ireland. The 1984 Conservative Party Conference was held in Brighton. Most of the party grandees, including senior leaders of the Tory Party from around the country, were staying at the Grand, a nine-storey, 178-room, Victorian hotel right on the seafront, which had just been refurbished. Virtually the entire Cabinet was staying there: the Prime Minister, Mrs Thatcher; Sir Geoffrey Howe, the Foreign Secretary; Leon Brittan, the Home Secretary; the Secretary of State for Education, Sir Keith Joseph; and the Health Minister, Norman Fowler. They had been to the Conference Ball on the Thursday night, which finished just after 1 o'clock in the morning. The bar closed at 2 o'clock and most people went off to bed, looking forward to the high point of the following day, the Leader's traditionally rousing speech on the Friday afternoon, 12 October.

Mrs Thatcher was in the Napoleon suite on the first floor, working on her speech; her husband, Denis, was in bed. At about 2.52a.m. she went to the bathroom, then returned to her desk. Two minutes later, at 2.54 there was a loud explosion as a bomb went off under the floorboards of room 629 on the sixth floor, right in the centre front of the hotel. The blast lifted the sixth and seventh floors up, then the accumulated rubble fell back on to the sixth floor, crashing downwards through room 629 where Gordon Shattock and his wife Jean were asleep. The debris fell through the front of the building which collapsed like a house of cards, through the fifth floor, where Eric Taylor and his wife Jennifer were asleep; the fourth-floor room below where John Wakeham, the Chief Whip and his wife Roberta were in bed; the third-floor room of Sir Anthony Berry and his wife Lady Sarah; and the second-floor room where Norman Tebbit and his wife Margaret were staying. Under Mr Tebbit's bedroom was the sitting room of the suite occupied by Sir Geoffrey Howe which was next to Mrs Thatcher's bathroom. The avalanche of debris fell between the two, into the main entrance below. Two minutes earlier and slightly to the right and it would have hit the Prime Minister.

The entrance of the hotel was suddenly filled with broken beams, sections of brickwork, carpets, furniture and swirling dust. Inside the lobby were most of the people from the five floors above, either trapped or dead. Those people nearby suffered a variety of injuries, including dust inhalation, and two police constables on duty in the entrance were seriously injured. The shock wave went right through the building but it was old and solid and most of the rest of the hotel remained intact. The corridors were soon filled with people, including police officers with guns drawn outside Mrs Thatcher's suite and standing guard at the windows.

At 2.56a.m. an emergency call went out from Brighton Police HQ: 'This is East Sussex; alert for major incident; act.'

Once the message had gone out, all the emergency services' telephone and radio networks went silent to give priority to organising the reaction to the bombing. The police put a cordon with a three-mile radius around the hotel with access restricted to emergency services' vehicles. At the East Sussex Ambulance HQ at Eastbourne the initiation of the major accident procedure was put into effect by sending two ambulances to the scene immediately and alerting others in the county that they might be needed. Senior ambulance officers were called at home and they went to the scene. In the meantime, the first crews to arrive reported back the need for further assistance. At the Royal Sussex County Hospital a system known as 'Cascade' was put into action to call up extra staff quickly; switchboard operators rang specified individuals at home, who in turn rang colleagues and so on until 100 extra staff were on their way to work in a matter of minutes. At the hospital, doctors began checking patients in the wards, deciding who could be moved to the lounges so that their beds could be made ready for bomb victims.

Back at the scene, by 3 o'clock the first ambulance arrived and the crew, once they had seen the devastation, called for ten more ambulances immediately. At 3.04, just ten minutes after the explosion, the first casualties, including the two injured police officers, were on their way to hospital.

Fire engines arrived outside the front of the hotel at 3.13 and fire fighters were the first into the building. Fireman David Norris, who was one of the first, met the Prime Minister coming out surrounded by Special Branch officers: 'Good morning,' she greeted him politely, 'I'm delighted to see you.' Mrs Thatcher was as unflustered as the emergency service personnel she met outside, saying to those she met as she climbed into her Jaguar: 'You read about these things happening but never believe it will happen to you.'

There was a gaping hole in the front of the building, and with the entrance blocked, staff and guests who were uninjured were evacuated through the fire escapes at the rear of the hotel. Inside there was the incessant ringing of fire alarms which made conversation, let alone listening for the injured, difficult, so firemen were detailed to smash them off the wall. Outside in the street, everybody who was there observed that a curious silence descended – no shouting, no crying, just clear orders and muted conversations.

Fortunately there was no fire since there was no gas main running through the hotel, but with 270 people in the hotel, the firemen radioed for six more fire engines. When Brighton's Chief Fire Officer, Fred Bishop, arrived shortly afterwards he called for another seven appliances, including two rescue tenders, to help people still trapped on the upper floors of the hotel. Three people were trapped on the seventh and eighth floors and the only way to rescue them was for three firemen to be hoisted up in a cradle suspended from a huge hydraulic arm, reach into the rubble and lift the victims out.

In the middle of the rescue operation, a suspected bomb was discovered in the Metropole Hotel nearby and it had to be evacuated too, adding to the load on the police.

The number of ambulances grew quickly, with crews coming from Hove, Lewes and Newhaven. Eventually a total of twenty ambulances started a ferry service, taking people with shock, dust inhalation, cuts and bruises and more serious injuries to the Royal Sussex, then returning with first-aid medical supplies, doctors – among them Dr David Bellamy – surgeons and paramedics to work on the site.

The main rescue task was in the hotel entrance where Fire Chief Fred Bishop and Fireman Tom McKinley began to examine the pile of rubble as soon as they arrived. They knew there were people alive once they heard a woman's voice from inside saying, 'Get me out.' It was difficult to know where to start, because going for one person might easily upset the balance of the collapsed building, bringing huge chunks of brickwork or timber down on them. It was also a race against time since the trapped people were obviously going to be injured.

Just below the entrance ceiling, Fred Bishop could see Norman Tebbit's feet sticking out of the rubble. Mr and Mrs Tebbit, though their room was lower down the building, finished up on top of Mr and Mrs Wakeham who had fallen further. Fred Bishop and Dr Bellamy and a team of firemen worked their way around the rubble and spoke to Mr Tebbit, from which they worked out that he was trapped close to his wife Margaret, both of them curled up in a foetal position under a mattress. They were surrounded by broken beams and one was resting across Mr Tebbit's back, and above that were tons of rubble. Both were conscious and Mr Tebbit wriggled to help the firemen move him, even though it caused great pain because he had a broken femur and had refused pain killers from Dr Bellamy. Dr Bellamy discovered that Mrs Tebbit had an injury to her neck. The doctor and other members of the team squeezed the Tebbits' hands to comfort them while they worked out the best way to extricate them. Once they had a plan, the firemen set to work with hacksaws to cut through the metal beams, using lifting gear and jacks to get them out, and filling buckets with rubble, then passing them along a human chain of firemen with the least disturbance since every time anybody moved it sent up clouds of dust. After a while, they managed to get water to moisten the Tebbits' lips. When Fred Bishop brushed against Mr Tebbit's feet and it hurt the feisty minister said, 'Get off my bloody feet, Fred.'

The main electricity cable had been cut, so the rescuers asked a BBC television crew to train their battery-powered lights on the scene. After three hours' work, at 5.44a.m. Mrs Tebbit was brought out, then an hour later, the firemen passed a stretcher into the pile of rubble and gently eased Mr Tebbit on to it and brought him out, passing him over their heads while the BBC camera team filmed it all for Breakfast Television. As soon as he was out he asked about his wife before an ambulanceman put an oxygen mask on his face. The rescuers struck up a strange rapport with Mr

Tebbit: he was among the first to praise them, but they made no secret of their admiration for him. The film of Mr Tebbit being lifted out by firemen, his face contorted with pain but through which he was still clearly still Norman Tebbit, the fiery, no-nonsense politician, was the memorable image of the whole rescue. Not only was his natural grit evident, but through it came his sense of humour too. He was admitted to the hospital at 7a.m. – four hours after the explosion – and when the admissions nurse asked him if he was allergic to anything he still had a joke: 'Yes,' he answered. 'Bombs.'

Once Mr and Mrs Tebbit were freed, the rescuers could attend to John and Roberta Wakeham. It took until 10.30 in the morning to free Mr Wakeham, the culmination of seven hours' work for he was the last person to be brought out alive. When the rescue team reached Mrs Wakeham she was dead. Sir Anthony Berry also died,

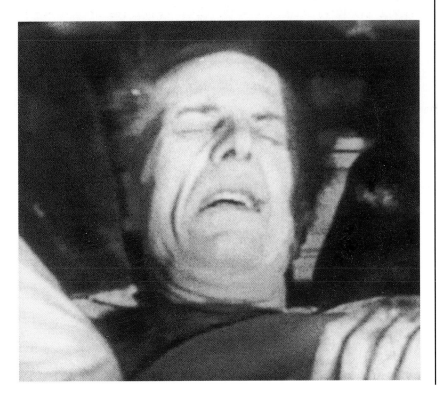

Norman Tebbit, MP, Secretary of State for Trade and Industry, being removed from the wreckage of the hotel's lobby after falling two floors; Mrs Margaret Tebbit suffered permanent injury in the blast.

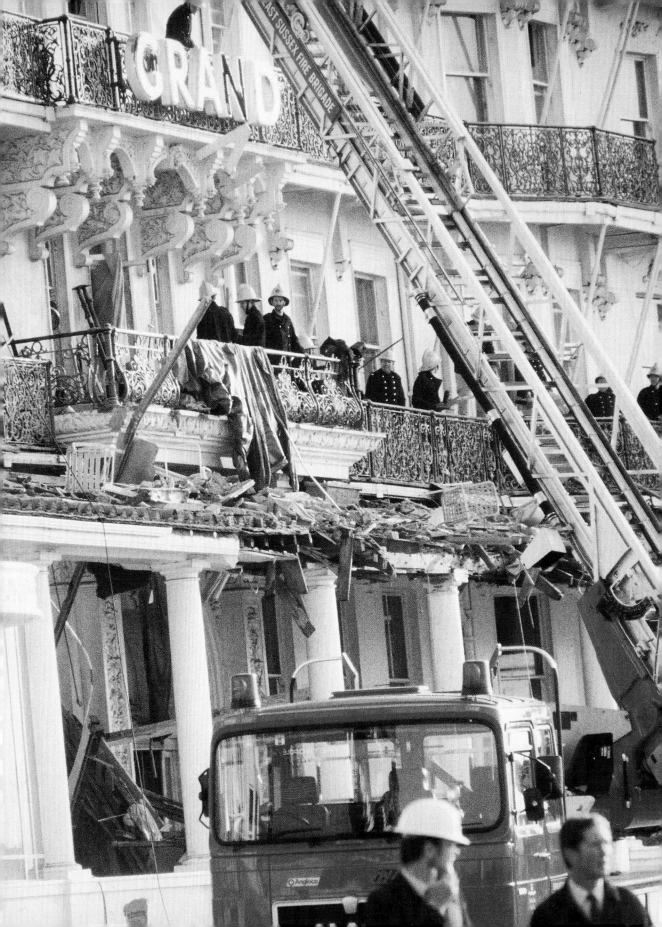

though his wife survived; Eric Taylor, who had fallen five floors, died, while his wife survived; Mrs Shattock died though her husband, who had fallen six floors, survived.

Strenuous efforts were made to make it business as usual at the Conference and they succeeded. The morning debate was on Northern Ireland, and it went ahead as planned. Douglas Hurd, the Northern Ireland Secretary, made no reference to the IRA.

At 11a.m. the major alert procedures were called off. At 11.20 the IRA claimed responsibility for the carnage, saying that its men had placed a 100lb gelignite bomb in the building. Mrs Thatcher visited the injured in hospital for an hour and a half before making her speech at 3p.m. to rapturous applause. The bombing, which could have been much more devastating and despite the tragedy of five deaths, was turned into something of a triumph for the government. Politicians had been at the receiving end of the emergency services' professionalism and it had certainly been something of a textbook operation from all three services, adding to the sense of triumph in adversity.

The bombing campaign continued, but public resolve seemed only to harden against giving in to terrorists. At Enniskillen on Remembrance Day 1987, a bomb at the war memorial service injured sixty-three people and eleven people were killed, including an off-duty nurse, Marie Wilson. In March 1993 at Warrington, a bomb in a litter bin in a shopping precinct killed two small boys; revulsion was the only emotion, but those killings gave renewed impetus to overtures for a ceasefire. On 1 August 1994 a ceasefire was agreed between the British and Irish governments, Sinn Fein and, indirectly, the IRA, bringing twenty-five years of terrorism to an uneasy halt. It had cost over 3000 people their lives. Clearly the civilian population of Northern Ireland, the armed forces and the police took the brunt of the casualties. However, the emergency services in general were in the front line of the hostilities and many

Opposite: The Grand Hotel, Brighton, 12 October 1984: firemen sifting through the wreckage following the explosion of an IRA bomb during the Conservative Party Conference which came close to wiping out the British government.

innocent people who might have died were saved, either by the vigilance or intervention of those services and the people prepared to occupy that front line in a purely humanitarian role.

In 1969, the same year that Northern Ireland erupted and the British Army was sent in, Yasser Arafat was appointed head of the Palestine Liberation Organisation (PLO). Four years later came the Yom Kippur War, putting back any resolution of the Arab–Israeli confrontation. In 1979, the Shah of Iran was overthrown by fundamentalist Islamic forces and the Iranian government held the entire staff of the US Embassy in Tehran hostage. Iran was convulsed by revolution, with different factions fighting for power in Tehran, adding to the potential for terrorism as more factions from the Middle East exported their terrorism on to the streets of European capitals.

On 30 April 1980, Police Constable Trevor Lock of the Metropolitan Police Diplomatic Patrol Group, a forty-one-year-old married man with three children, was on guard duty outside the Iranian Embassy in Princes Gate, overlooking Hyde Park. He was armed, but his pistol was concealed inside his uniform.

At 11.30a.m., three Iranians approached the Embassy. One of them went up to Lock who realised too late that they were armed terrorists and did not have time to draw his gun. He took on the first man, but they grabbed him and fired their guns at the windows, sending glass flying, then pushed Lock through the front door. Three more terrorists arrived and they quickly overpowered the guards inside, injuring one of the Iranian staff in the process. The Ambassador tried to escape by jumping out of a window into the rear courtyard, but the gunmen found him and brought him back. They then went through the whole five-storey building, taking everybody hostage. There were eighteen Iranian diplomats, three other Iranian nationals and five British citizens, including two BBC TV news journalists, Christopher Cramer and Sim Harris, who were in the Embassy to apply for visas to go to Iran to cover the upheaval.

One of the diplomats managed to set off an alarm which was linked to Scotland Yard and within minutes the first armed police had arrived outside. The terrorists had taken Lock's personal radio, and police on the operation had to be issued with new radios which operated on frequencies which it could not pick up.

The police established contact with the gunmen first by shouting through an open window, then by telephone which the terrorists used to make their demands: the release of ninety-one political prisoners being held in an oil-rich, partly Arab-speaking province of Iran, Khuzestan, which they called Arabistan; and an aircraft to fly them out of the country. If the Iranian government did not comply, then they said they would kill the hostages within twenty-four hours. Their leader, 'Salim', used the telephone to speak to the Iranian Foreign Minister who was on a visit to Abu Dhabi. Iranian journalists who were with the minister heard him say that if one drop of blood was spilt, the same number of prisoners would be tried and executed.

Outside, the police operation was bolstered by trained negotiators, a psychiatrist, Arab and Farsi translators and more armed police who cordoned off the whole area, then evacuated the adjoining buildings, including a number of other embassies. Police marksmen took up positions at key points at the front and the rear of the building. The terrorists asked for a doctor for the injured diplomat, then in a telex to the BBC, the leader of the group apologised to the British people for the hostage taking and claimed that the police had refused to send in a doctor.

The police were activating a well-rehearsed plan for dealing with sieges which had been built on the experience gained from the IRA Balcombe Street siege. The Special Air Service was put on standby

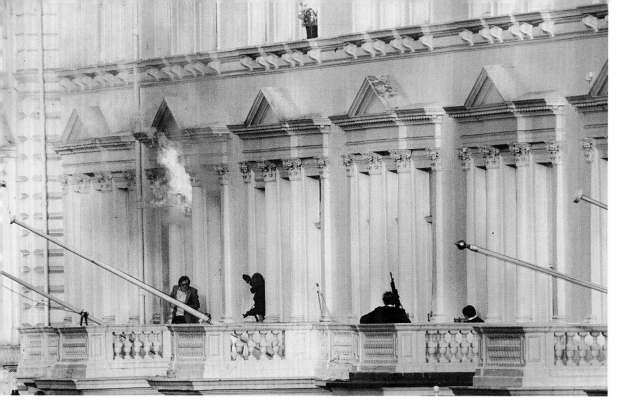

Princes Gate, London, 30 April 1980: SAS troopers storming the Iranian Embassy to end the siege by gunmen who had just killed one of the diplomats; the figure escaping from the fire (extreme left) is Sim Harris, a BBC journalist.

in case offensive action was needed and the whole operation came under the control of the Home Secretary, William Whitelaw. The basis of the plan was to be patient rather than confrontational, to wear down the terrorists' will to go on by constant firm but friendly negotiation and by controlling the supply of food to chip away at their morale.

The policy paid some small dividends immediately: a young girl was released on the first evening; another hostage the following day; then two more on the Friday, including the BBC's Christopher Cramer. On the Saturday, a sick man was released and a pregnant woman, Mrs Haj Deah Kanji. One of the released hostages brought out a letter from Trevor Lock which told the police that if there was an assault, he would go for the leader of the group.

The international media circus which had arrived and set up camp outside the police cordon in Hyde Park expanded daily as the tension rose, with literally thousands of cameras – television and press – trained on the front of the building. With the eyes of the world watching the crisis, a group of Iranian students gathered at the police cordon, demonstrating against the terrorists' action.

Over the telephone the gunmen demanded that the ambassadors of Algeria, Jordan and other Arab countries be brought in to negotiate the release of the hostages and the terrorists' safe conduct out of the country, but the police stalled the move, saying that the ambassadors would not act as go-betweens and that no country would give them asylum even if an aircraft was made available.

The police stayed in control but in the background members of the SAS Regiment were preparing for an assault. They had been standing by at the Balcombe Street siege, but had not been needed, but if the building had to be taken by force, they had skills and equipment the police did not have. The technique of installing listening devices and mini-cameras into the building from adjoining buildings to create a picture of what was going on inside went on as quietly as possible, but inside the Embassy the gunmen heard the

Rear view: SAS men abseiling down the back of the Iranian Embassy building; the whole action lasted eleven minutes in which five terrorists died and only one survived to face trial.

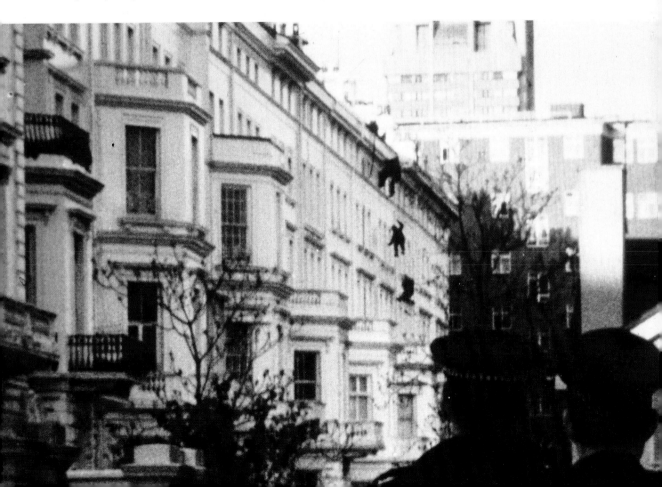

drilling noises which added to their anxiety. Trevor Lock convinced them that the noises were made by faulty water pipes or mice. In fact, the soldiers were removing bricks from the wall leaving only a layer of plaster to burst through if they had to attack.

The tension inside the building rose steadily. On the Sunday afternoon, members of the Embassy staff asked the gunmen to clean off anti-Khomeini slogans which they had daubed on the walls. Mr Labasani, the press attaché, was particularly argumentative and one of the gunmen, called Faisal, rushed across the room. Trevor Lock moved into his path and held his arm against the gunman and the confrontation died down. The fracas led the gunman to notice that there was a bulge in one of the walls which he said had previously been flat when he wrote the slogans on it.

On Sunday evening, a Syrian journalist, Mustapha Karkouti, was released suffering from acute stomach pains and he was taken away in an ambulance. In reality, the gunmen were running out of patience: they had set deadlines which had been ignored; they had not been allowed to speak to Arab ambassadors; and there seemed little possibility of a negotiated settlement. They became more unstable according to later police reports, expecting an attack. On the Monday afternoon, 5 May, they said they would execute a hostage every half an hour unless their demands were met. They had made similar threats before, but this time at 1.15p.m. they carried them out, a number of shots being heard. The gunmen killed Mr Abbas Labasani, the diplomat who had volunteered himself to be the first to die.

Hearing the shots, the Metropolitan Police Commissioner, Sir David McNee, wrote a letter explaining that in Britain the police enforced the law and that he and his officers could not give in, but that if they gave up, the men would be treated properly; they had nothing to fear.

At 6.40p.m., more shots were heard, then fifteen minutes later

Mr Labasani's body was dumped on the Embassy doorstep. Police started talking positively over the telephone about the possibility of transport, but the gunmen only became more agitated, expecting an assault. They were right: after consulting with the Home Secretary, Sir David McNee handed over responsibility for the siege to a senior Army officer in a letter timed at 7.07p.m. At 7.15, a series of explosions shook the building and a fire started on the second floor where the SAS had managed to place charges against the outside of the windows to blow them in; they also threw in stun grenades. SAS troopers climbed through the windows as smoke started pouring from the building and the sound of gunfire inside the building was clear. Television cameras went into action and normal programmes were interrupted as the assault was broadcast round the world live.

Inside the building, the gunmen opened fire on the Iranian hostages, killing one and badly wounding another. As they did so, Trevor Lock took out his gun, which the gunmen had never searched for, and tackled the leader of the group as he said he would. When the SAS arrived, a trooper separated them and shot 'Salim' dead.

The troopers moved through the building at speed, killing five of the gunmen; the sixth hid among the Iranian women hostages and gave up when he was identified by one of the SAS men. One gunman and nineteen hostages were taken alive from the Embassy to hospital, some of them injured, some of them unconscious, but all survived.

As soon the SAS operation was complete, control was handed back to the police. The success of the assault was remarkable and a testimony to the skills of the SAS, but the men who carried it out disappeared quickly after the operation, keen to preserve their anonymity. The surviving gunman was sentenced to life imprisonment with a recommendation that he serve at least thirty years.

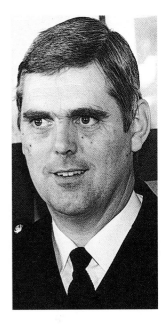

The hero of the Iranian Embassy siege, PC Trevor Lock of the Metropolitan Police Diplomatic Protection Squad, managed to keep his gun hidden throughout the siege and tackled the terrorist leader as the SAS attacked.

Constable Trevor Lock, who had acted with extraordinary judgement and courage throughout the siege, returned to duty a month later, and on 30 June he was given the Freedom of the City of London. He was later awarded the George Cross.

A constant feature of the Iranian siege was the presence of groups of Iranian 'students', both anti-Khomeini and pro-Khomeini factions, chanting protests which would not have been allowed in their own country. On 17 April 1984, a group of young Libyans had planned a demonstration outside the Libyan Embassy in St James's Square – or the 'Peoples' Bureau' as the Libyans described it. They were marching to protest against the Libyan ruler, Colonel Gaddafi, who had hanged two students in public in the grounds of Tripoli University. Libyan politics had been a source of concern for the police for some time following reports of Libyan 'hit squads' being sent to seek out opponents of the Gaddafi regime in Britain and kill them. Gaddafi was determined to stop the demonstration and the night before it was to take place two Libyan diplomats went to the Foreign Office and told the night officer that there could be a violent response from the Bureau if it went ahead. The Libyan diplomats then engaged two television crews from UP/ITN to cover the demonstration.

The police arrived in St James's Square in the early morning, preparing the route and erecting barriers to keep the marchers away from a small pro-Gaddafi demonstration made up of people from the Bureau which had gathered outside it. Just after 10 o'clock the main demonstration of about seventy people, their heads covered in masks, came through the square. A line of five police officers stood in the centre of the road between the two groups. Loud music was blaring from the Bureau to drown the chants of the anti-Gaddafi protesters. Suddenly a window on the first floor of the Bureau opened and a sub-machine gun was poked through. There was a ten-second burst of fire into the crowd which scattered leaving eleven people injured where they lay. Among them in the middle of the road was a young policewoman, Yvonne Fletcher, who had been shot through the stomach.

Armed policemen took up firing positions in the square as unarmed officers, including WPC Fletcher's fiancé, PC Michael Liddle, rushed to her side and gave her first aid. Ambulances arrived swiftly and one crew carried her to the side of the road then into an ambulance under cover from the armed policemen. The ambulance took her to the Westminster Hospital where surgeons started working to save her life.

Police cars with more armed officers rushed to the scene and a police helicopter equipped with a video camera was called in to hover over out of range. The surrounding buildings were cleared – in some cases it meant police taking people out through the roof to keep them away from the firing line in front of the building. Behind the Embassy, a policeman threw a jacket over the Libyans' own security camera so they could not see what the police were doing. Around the square the police were putting into practice all that had been learned from previous sieges. First, they established a cordon around the area patrolled by sixty officers, all of them well out of the line of fire. Then they moved on to the surrounding rooftops, putting up sandbag emplacements at suitable vantage points for marksmen from the D.11 Specialist Armed Unit. They were equipped with rifles which had image intensifiers and night vision.

The police laid siege to the Embassy, but this time the occupants were not holding anybody hostage. It was simply that among them there was a murderer who enjoyed diplomatic immunity from arrest, because just after midday it had been announced from the hospital that Yvonne Fletcher was dead.

The Home Secretary, Leon Brittan, took charge, moving to the Cabinet Office Briefing Room – known as COBRA – a room specially set up for the management of crises which had also been used

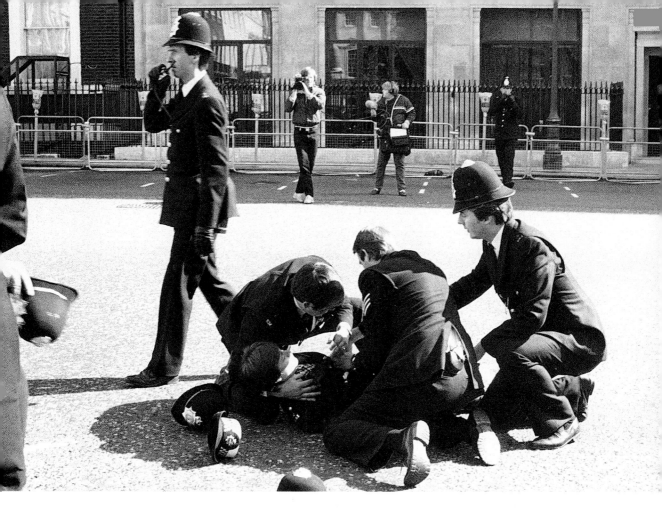

Police officers rush to the side of WPC Yvonne Fletcher after she was hit by a burst of fire from a sub-machine gun from inside the Libyan Embassy.

during the Iranian siege. He demanded that the Bureau be checked for arms and explosives and that the forty diplomats leave the building to be questioned by the police. The Bureau staff refused to move and they denied any part in the shooting, saying that the shots must have come from somebody in the crowd.

In Tripoli, Colonel Gaddafi took charge, telephoning his Bureau regularly with new instructions. With memories of the highly successful police and SAS operation in storming the Iranian Embassy, Gaddafi was immediately worried that Britain would use similar tactics again. A series of rambling statements was issued via the Libyan News Agency, Jana, accusing Britain of attacking the Bureau 'in the most ugly form of terrorist attack'. On the ground, he took a more practical step by using Libyan 'revolutionary guards' to surround the British Embassy in Tripoli, effectively turning the ambassador and his staff into hostages.

In St James's Square police activity intensified: huge blue plastic screens were erected around a large white van which was a control centre linked to all the electronic aids which are the eyes and ears of the police. Highly sensitive, directional microphones were set up on nearby rooftops as were video cameras, all trained on the exterior of the Bureau. Generators and powerful lights were set up in case the Libyans tried anything at night. Police are rightly cagey about revealing all their equipment and methods, but there is little doubt they would have found ways to drill through the walls from neighbouring buildings to place mini-microphones, the sound of drilling apparently masked by aircraft. On the first night, a military aircraft did make three passes over the area of central London, an unusual place for the RAF to fly. An SAS team was brought in case it was needed.

On Sunday, the British government announced that diplomatic relations with Libya would be severed and the occupants of the Bureau had seven days to leave Britain. The following Sunday was set for their departure, and for the British Embassy staff to return from Tripoli.

Throughout the siege, there was a poignant reminder for everybody of what had happened: Yvonne Fletcher's hat, surrounded by those of the officers who had rushed to her side after the shooting, lay unrecovered in the road, a symbol of sadness and courage. On the Friday, the day before Yvonne Fletcher's funeral, a police officer in a flak jacket went into the square and retrieved it. The following day, Yvonne Fletcher was buried after a service which packed Salisbury Cathedral. Six hundred police officers travelled from London to Wiltshire, as did the Home Secretary and the Metropolitan Police Commissioner. Her coffin was draped in the Metropolitan Police flag and on top of it rested her hat. The death

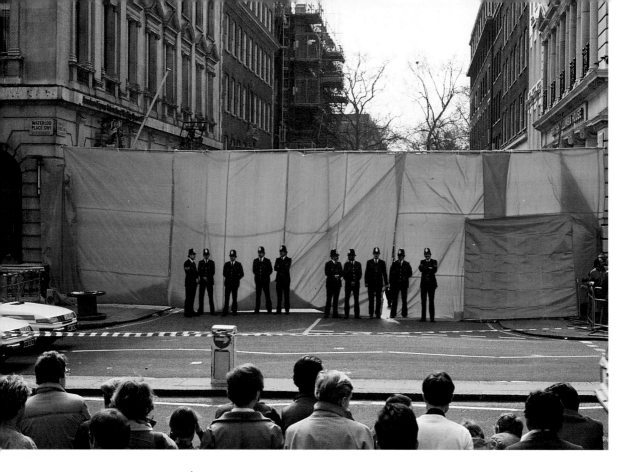

Libyan Embassy, St James's Square, 17 April 1984: police sealed off the square with screens to obscure their operations after a burst of gunfire from the Embassy killed a police officer.

of an unarmed young woman on duty at a demonstration which had nothing to do with Britain disgusted the British public and brought out mixed emotions – of pride certainly, but also of hopelessness that despite a superb police operation, WPC Fletcher's murderer was about to escape.

With the siege in St James's Square under control, suddenly Middle Eastern politics erupted in Kensington when Iranian students opposed to Ayatollah Khomeini invaded the Iranian Consulate in concert with similar actions in capitals all over Europe. There was fighting with the consular staff, but the demonstrators were confined to the ground floor as the staff retreated behind a security door. The police routine was soon in full swing, as they sealed off the area, erected screens and placed armed police officers at key points, some of them straight from the Libyan Embassy. But the incident ended peacefully when the consular staff

114

released the students one by one, their hands tied behind their backs.

The following day, the British Embassy staff in Tripoli were released and flown to Britain, triggering the arrival of coaches outside the Libyan Bureau to take the diplomats and their families, 140 people in all, to Heathrow and back to Tripoli.

The siege had lasted ten days. There had been no more bloodshed, but it had left a nasty feeling among the police. In the police magazine *The Job*, Sir Kenneth Newman summed it up: 'We can all draw some small satisfaction from knowing that Yvonne Fletcher's untimely death has resulted in the expulsion from this country of people who posed a threat to the safety of our citizens. But let me not fudge the issue. With every other police officer, I would like to have had the satisfaction of an arrest.'

Yvonne Fletcher's death sparked off a wave of revulsion at the very idea that Middle Eastern countries could use London's streets to settle their differences. It was not for British police officers to die in that way. That feeling manifested itself in the Police Memorial Trust which was formed at the instigation of the film director Michael Winner to erect memorials to officers who died in the course of duty. The first memorial of Portland stone was erected where Yvonne Fletcher had fallen. The ceremony was attended by the Prime Minister and the Leader of the Opposition. In September 1985, the Trust erected a memorial to the three police officers who had died in Hans Crescent in the Harrods bombing on 18 December 1982.

As the terror campaigns generated from Ireland and the Middle East have shown, bombing innocent people does not achieve very much – if anything it only stiffens the resolve to resist the bombers' demands. Terrorism lasted twenty-five years in Ireland until the current ceasefire and in Palestine the first tentative steps towards peace are being taken. The security measures taken to counter those campaigns remain in place since other groups with ideological or

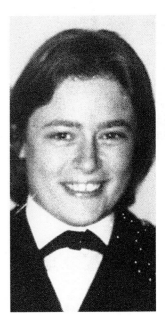

WPC Yvonne Joyce Fletcher, aged twenty-five, had been in the police force for seven years when she was murdered by an unknown gunman from the Libyan Embassy.

religious motives continue to resort to violence. The lethal gas attack in Japan on Tokyo's underground in January 1995 which killed twelve people and injured hundreds, and the bomb at the US Federal Government building in Oklahoma in April 1995 which killed 167 people and injured many more, show how the tactics of the bomber and the maimer will still be used within a society as well as from outside. For the foreseeable future, police forces and rescue service workers will have to put their lives on the line.

The police, while coping with international terrorism, have always had to face a wide variety of dangerous circumstances from criminals, political agitators and deranged people in Britain. They need to be ready for such circumstances as and when they happen. Sometimes though, an incident is simply impossible to plan for, and what happened on Wednesday 19 August 1987 in the sleepy market town of Hungerford in Berkshire was just such an incident.

At 12.40p.m. there was a 999 call to Thames Valley Police from a motorcyclist who had witnessed an extraordinary scene at the Golden Arrow filling station on the A4 at Froxfield, just to the west of Hungerford. A man armed with an assault rifle had attacked the filling station kiosk, firing a shot through the window at the cashier. Two minutes later there was a second 999 call, this time to Wiltshire police, from the cashier, Mrs Kakoub Dean, to say that she had been shot at by a gunman, but that his gun had run out of ammunition and he had driven off towards Hungerford in a Vauxhall Astra GTE.

The Thames Valley Police Tactical Firearms Team could not be deployed immediately because it was on a training exercise at an Army firing range and had to be recalled first. The police helicopter – one of only four in the country in 1987 – which could have been used to search for the gunman was undergoing minor repairs, so it would be delayed. Three police cars, none of them with armed police inside, responded to the call and began to look for the Astra. Even as they began to search, a radio message came through to say that another 999 call had been made from a woman in South View, a street in Hungerford, to report another shooting which was believed to be linked to the incident at Froxfield.

Before long, the radio network was alive with reports of shootings in Hungerford, but hard information about exactly what had happened was difficult to sift out from the huge number of reports. Over the congested radio, the three unarmed traffic policemen devised a plan. South View was a cul-de-sac, one end opening on to Fairview Road, which ran parallel to Hungerford High Street, while the other end opened out on to Hungerford Common. They decided that PC Roger Brereton would go to the junction between South View and Fairview Road, while the other two would drive over the Common to the other end of the cul-de-sac, sealing off the road. As PC Brereton was arriving at South View, a general call went out over the radio from police headquarters advising all officers to be cautious; the latest information was that the gunman had injured somebody else. In fact it was infinitely worse than that.

Michael Ryan lived at 4 South View with his mother, Dorothy Ryan, who doted on him. He was twenty-seven and he had lived there all his life. He was a spoilt child with few friends; he was a loner, a fantasist and a gun fanatic. He was a member of a local gun club where he practised with his collection of guns, all held completely legally: three pistols; a Second World War American M.1 rifle; and the pride of his collection, a Chinese copy of the famous Russian AK-47 Kalashnikov semi-automatic assault rifle.

As PC Brereton turned into South View, Ryan opened fire on the police car with the Kalashnikov and a Beretta 9mm pistol. The policeman was hit four times, but he managed to make a single call asking for assistance and telling his control that he had been shot before he collapsed into the passenger seat and died.

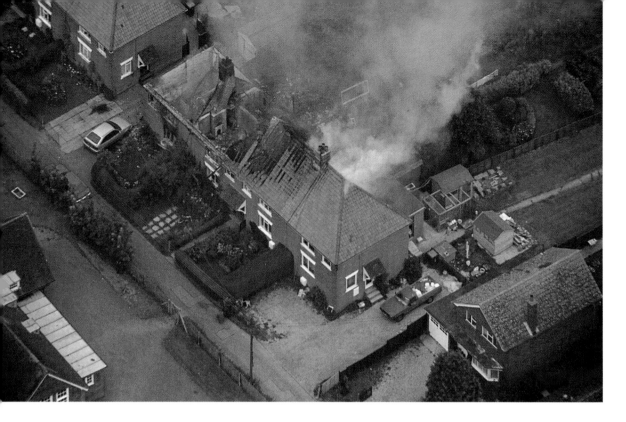

South View, Hungerford, 19 August 1987: before setting out on his murderous rampage through the town, Michael Ryan set his own home on fire; the semi-detached house was rebuilt as a single, detached house.

Roger Brereton was Michael Ryan's fifth victim that day. His murderous rampage had started before the attack on the filling station when he had murdered Mrs Sue Godfrey in the Savernake Forest, shooting her several times in the back with the Kalashnikov while her children, with whom she had just had a picnic, waited in the car for her. He had tried to kill Mrs Dean in the filling station, but had run out of ammunition and her life was spared. He then went to his home, collected some survival gear, then set fire to his mother's house. When his car refused to start, he fired several shots at it before turning on a neighbour, Mr Roland Mason, who was painting his fence, killing him with six shots. Then he killed Mr Mason's wife, Sheila, at the back of the house with a single shot. Another neighbour, Mrs Margery Jackson, was in the window of her house and Ryan fired at her, wounding her but not fatally. She phoned her husband at work to tell him what had happened.

Ryan then set off towards the Common, shooting a fourteen-year-old girl in her doorway and seriously injuring her, then killing

Mr Ken Clements who was out for a walk with his family. Then he turned and went back up South View to the T junction with Priory Road at the other end where he shot at a car driven by Linda Chapman with her daughter Allison. Both were wounded, but Mrs Chapman had the presence of mind to drive away quickly to the doctor's surgery for treatment. It was then that PC Brereton turned the corner and Ryan shot him. Next he went down Priory Road, where he saw Mr Abdul Rahman Khan mowing his lawn. Ryan took careful aim and shot him too.

At the other end of South View, PC Jeremy Wood had arrived in his car just as Ryan headed back into South View from Priory Road and started shooting at him. PC Wood had seen Ken Clements' body and he called on the radio asking for armed assistance, then started clearing people from the Common. By this time, ambulances were on their way to South View, the first one driven by Linda Bright with her colleague Hazel Haslett. As they arrived, Ryan opened fire on them and they had to drive away at speed having reported that they had come under fire.

Ryan's next victim was George White, a friend of the Jackson family who had offered to drive Ivor Jackson home from work to see his wife who had been injured. As they arrived, Ryan raked the car killing George White and seriously injuring Ivor Jackson, the car crashing into PC Brereton's. Dorothy Ryan arrived home from shopping to be confronted with the carnage which her son was creating in the street. She walked down South View and called to Michael to stop shooting, but he turned the gun on her and killed her with two shots, then set off across the Common.

Police starting setting up road blocks to keep people away from Ryan, but nobody knew where he was. At 1.08, half an hour after the first 999 call, the Tactical Firearms Team was ordered to go to Hungerford, but it would take time to get there. In the meantime, two armed officers whose normal duties were with the Diplomatic

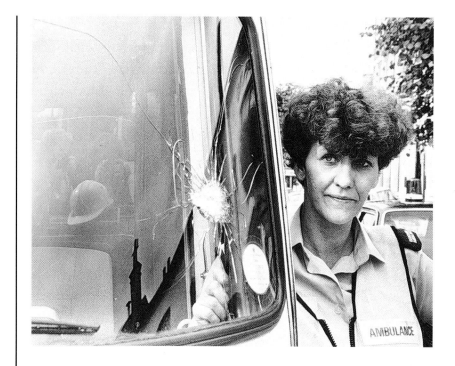

Linda Bright, of the Berkshire Ambulance service, shows where a bullet from Michael Ryan's AK-47 damaged the windscreen of her ambulance when she drove into South View to attend to some of his earlier victims. Her colleague Hazel Haslett was injured by Ryan.

Protection Squad arrived just before 1.30p.m. They were armed with pistols only and took up positions on the Common, but Ryan had moved away from South View and was now on the other side of the Common where his next victim, Francis Butler, was out walking his dog. He shot him, then moved on.

An off-duty air stewardess, Carol Hall, was at the swimming pool close to where Francis Butler had been shot. She heard the firing and reported it to the pool manager, Michael Palmer, and to David Sparrow, a lifeguard, and they went outside and saw Butler's body and Ryan close by. They evacuated the swimmers, mostly children, to the changing rooms.

Outside, a taxi driver, Mr Marcus Barnard, was driving home past the pool. Ryan saw the car and shot him through the windscreen. With great courage, Carol Hall, Michael Palmer and David Sparrow went to his aid, but he was dead. The next victim was John Storms, a washing machine engineer who was parking his van in order to start a job at a nearby house as Ryan shot him. Hearing the shots, a builder, Bob Barclay, dashed out and dragged Storms into the house, just as Ryan started shooting at another car, killing Douglas Wainwright who was driving to see his son, a Hungerford policeman. As cars came down the street, so Ryan shot the drivers – first Eric Vardy who was driving home, then Sandra Hill whose car crashed after she had been hit. An off-duty soldier, Lance-Corporal Carl Harries, heard the shooting and came out to see what was going on. He went to the crashed car to see if he could do anything for her and as he was caring for her he heard more shots.

Ryan had forced his way into the home of Victor Gibbs and his wife Myrtle by shooting off the lock. He killed Victor Gibbs with one shot as he tried to protect his wife by throwing himself in front of her wheelchair. Leaving them in the kitchen, Ryan then started firing from the house, injuring some people, but killing Ian Playle and injuring his wife. They had already been turned away at one police road block and were looking for an alternative route through Hungerford when Ryan fired on their car. Carl Harries attended to them all, giving comfort and providing what first aid he could.

In a orgy of killing lasting less than two hours, Ryan had killed sixteen people without apparent motive. His erratic progress through the town made it very difficult for the rescue services to find his victims but by 2.15p.m., ambulances had managed to pick up some of the dead and wounded and they started taking them to the Princess Margaret Hospital some fifteen miles from Hungerford.

Consciously or not, Ryan was making his way towards the John O'Gaunt Comprehensive School where he had been a student ten years previously. On the way he shot George Noon in the head, leaving him lying injured in his garden. At this point, the police

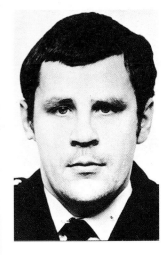

PC Roger Brereton, who was shot dead by Michael Ryan as he turned into South View in his police car to investigate the reported shootings.

helicopter arrived overhead with a marksman on board armed with a shotgun. It was no match for the Kalashnikov, so once the policeman heard how Ryan was armed, he landed and picked up a rifle, then continued the search, but failed to see any sign of Ryan.

The Tactical Firearms Team also arrived under the command of Sergeant Paul Brightwell. They changed into their protective clothing in the town and drew their weapons at 2.20. They started searching the town on foot while other policemen in armoured Land Rovers drove through the town, picking up wounded where they could. The search took most of the afternoon, as they gradually worked their way through the town towards the school where they spotted Ryan at a window at 5.26p.m. They quickly closed in and surrounded the building. That meant that the rest of Hungerford could be declared safe and rescue work could continue without danger.

Brightwell tried to negotiate with Ryan for over an hour, but to no avail; just before 7 o'clock Ryan turned a pistol on himself in one of the first-floor classrooms and shot himself in the head.

There were criticisms of the police reaction to the shooting, some of them directed at the armed officers on the Common who stayed where they were. An inquiry was set up, but it did not blame the police. As senior officers pointed out, nobody knew where Ryan was; nobody knew where to go; there were tens of thousands of telephone calls in the space of that hour; and the sheer volume of calls had created confusion on the ground.

There was no doubt that some people had behaved with great courage, and the Queen's Commendation for Brave Conduct was awarded posthumously to PC Roger Brereton, and to PC Jeremy Wood and ambulancewomen Linda Bright and Hazel Haslett, who continued to pick up and tend to the injured during the afternoon. Carol Hall, Michael Palmer, David Sparrow and Lance-Corporal Carl Harries were also awarded the medal.

It was by far and away the worst case of shooting in British criminal history and one which nobody could have anticipated. There were calls for arming the police, but in general the police resisted that call, preferring instead to push for ever-tighter controls on the availability of such weapons as Ryan had and could own quite legally.

The Hungerford massacre has so far been a one-off, the action of a single, deranged man acting out some kind of fantasy. In June 1982, another deranged gunman, Barry Prudom, killed two police officers in Harrogate before turning the gun on himself, but such incidents are rare, if devastating when they do happen, and the police have to be constantly aware that they could.

There is a huge difference between madmen and criminals, but the number of occasions on which criminals have been prepared to use weapons has steadily increased over the last two decades. Between 1980 and 1993, thirty-two police officers have lost their lives and many more been seriously injured in the course of duty,

Frontline Britain: riots in city centres and poor housing estates have become a regular feature of police work in the 1980s and 1990s, and it is police officers who have had to face increasingly hostile and often violent elements in a more divided society.

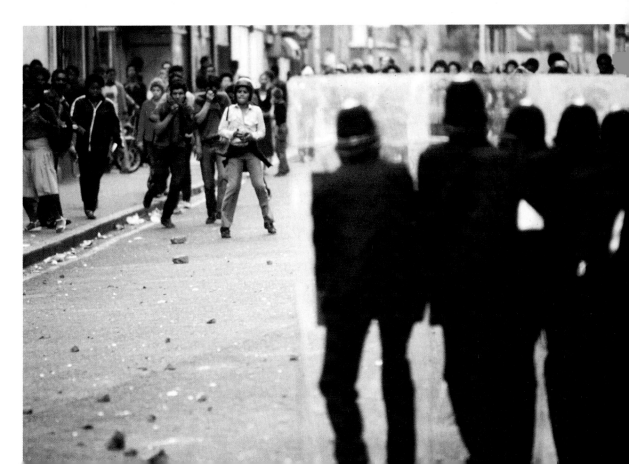

with deaths in every year except 1986. Many of them were killed in armed raids on banks, but some were killed in trivial circumstances, such as Sergeant Michael Hawcroft who was stabbed to death by a youth suspected of car theft; WPC Mandy Rayner, aged eighteen, who was killed in a row following a breath test in Royston, Hertfordshire; Sergeant Ross Hunt who was stabbed to death attending a pub brawl in Lanarkshire; and Special Constable Glenn Goodman who was shot dead by the IRA on a routine vehicle check near Tadcaster in Yorkshire.

Many police officers have tackled armed men and lived. On 15 October 1992, Detective Constables Stephen Thomas and Alan Knapp tackled armed raiders as they were robbing a Post Office, shooting them both and seriously injuring them; both were awarded the George Medal. Two weeks later, Detective Sergeant Robert Window went to a flat in Tottenham with a search warrant. The occupier of the flat went for him with a sword and cut his hand off. Neighbours packed his severed hand in frozen food and sent it with Sergeant Window in the HEMS air ambulance which took him to the Vernon Hospital in Northwood where it was sewn back on with micro-surgery.

There have always been armed criminals but the trend is growing, and armed men, especially those involved in the illegal drugs trade, are increasingly prepared to kill anybody who gets in their way, especially police officers. The clearest example of the cultural clash between the traditional, quiet, non-confrontational type of policing Britain has enjoyed for 170 years and the modern, ruthless, professional, armed criminal came on 20 October 1993 in South London. A 999 call to Clapham police station at 8.10p.m. described a domestic dispute going on in Cato Road. PC Patrick Dunne, a community policeman and a single man aged forty-four, went by bicycle to investigate. He arrived in the road and made inquiries, and while he was talking to two men in the doorway of a house, he heard shots from across the street. He pushed the men inside for safety and walked towards the house just as three men ran out waving guns. One of them pointed a gun at him and fired from about thirty feet as PC Dunne approached them, hitting him on the right side of his chest. The men then ran off laughing.

Police cars and ambulances were quickly on the scene, but PC Dunne was dead. So was the occupier of the house who had been murdered by the men as part of a turf war between rival drugs gangs. Police closed off a large area of Clapham, including the High Street, and a police helicopter arrived overhead, but the suspects managed to escape the cordon.

PC Patrick Dunne's death was felt deeply by the community he served. There were warm tributes to him from all parts of that community when he was buried in Clapham. Those tributes came from people who want the idea of unarmed policing by consent to continue as the basis of policing in Britain. The feeling that police should not be armed routinely is deeply embedded in British life, but it is becoming difficult to sustain in inner city areas where drug dealers especially frequently carry guns, first to protect the areas in which they carry on their illegal trade, but also to use against the police and the other emergency services to avoid arrest.

There is a new frontline developing in Britain. It threads its way along city streets and around poor housing estates, an invisible dividing line between a wary police force and an increasingly alienated section of society, the underclass. In most big cities there are well-defined, run-down areas where most people live in relative poverty, at the bottom of what they see as a winner–loser society. A semi-outlaw society has developed in neighbourhoods where the illegal drugs business thrives and where violence perpetrated by armed gangs which have grown up to protect it is commonplace. It has reached the point where policing some areas has become so dangerous that even ambulance crews in Moss Side, Manchester,

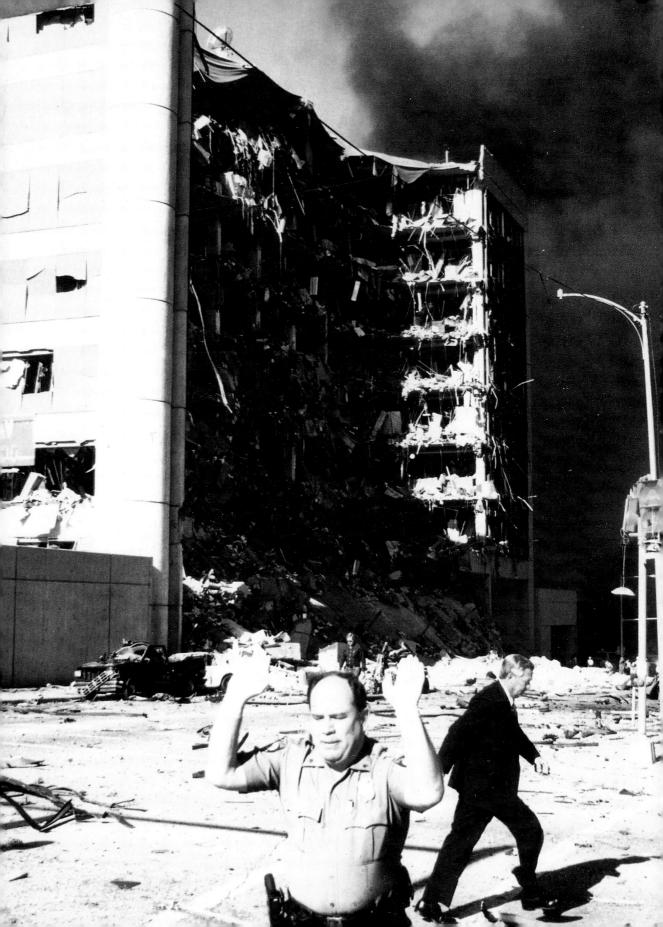

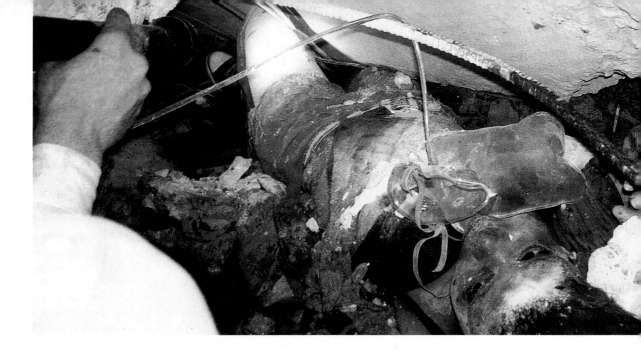

for example, wear flak jackets when they are called to patients in the area.

These problems will not be solved by arming the police. Shootouts on street corners will not stop drug dealing; that will take careful legislation, social policies and expenditure designed to break down the divisions in society which riots, such as those in Manningham in Bradford, Toxteth in Liverpool and Chapeltown in Leeds, have so clearly shown exist. The police can only contain the situation until social solutions to those problems can be found.

Above: Rescuers worked in extremely dangerous conditions in the Oklahoma bombing to reach those trapped in the rubble. Here, Diana Bradley is trapped by her leg which surgeons later amputated on the spot to release her.

Opposite: Frontline America: the Federal Government building in Oklahoma City was devastated by a huge car bomb on 19 April 1995, allegedly planted by extreme right-wing terrorists, killing over 200 people.

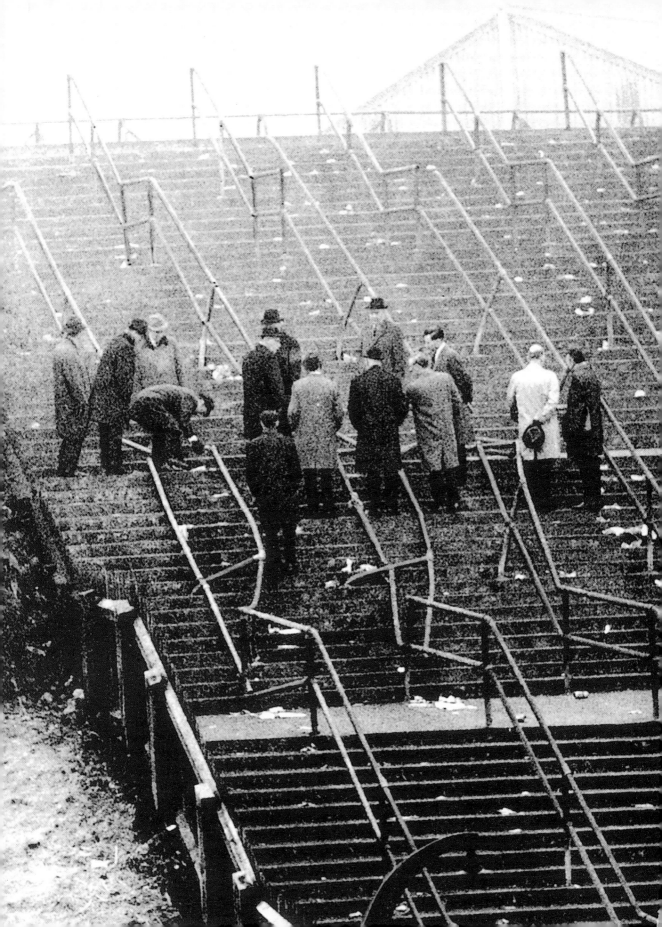

Chapter Five

FOOTBALL – A QUESTION FOR SPORT

Football stadia are the modern equivalents of amphitheatres – places for sport, entertainment and atmosphere, places to let go, to be emotional and to be fiercely partisan. It is a great, slightly dangerous feeling to stand in the tightly packed terraces with upwards of 35,000 other people, everybody roaring and swaying as one in support of a team, looking forward to the final rush of excitement which comes with winning.

But the excitement which goes with football matches can also bring danger. Many grounds are old and improvements in the facilities, especially in the provision of built-in safety measures, have lagged behind the huge growth in the sport since the war. Since then people have had greater mobility to get to away matches and the game has become more partisan. A major part of the problem was the tradition of standing on the terraces where barriers help to break up the crowd, but controlling tens of thousands of people surging for entrances and exits, or high on excitement during and especially after the match has always been a huge problem for the police and for the clubs. In 1902, the worst football crowd disaster happened at Glasgow Rangers' Ibrox Stadium when part of the terracing collapsed, killing twenty-five people and injuring 517. In 1946, it was surpassed when a barrier in the terracing gave way

Opposite: Ibrox Stadium, Glasgow: officials examine the twisted barriers on Staircase 13 following a match between Rangers and Celtic on 2 January 1971 when fans tumbled down it, killing sixty-six people.

under crowd pressure in the Bolton versus Stoke Cup Tie and thirty-three people died and over 500 were injured.

On Saturday 2 January 1971, Glasgow had been stirring from early on for the high point of the football calendar in Scotland – the New Year fixture between Glasgow Rangers and Glasgow Celtic to be played at Ibrox. There was no score and the match had been frustrating for both sides right up to the last minute, when Celtic did score, giving them virtually a certain victory. Rangers fans, believing that it was over, began to leave before the final whistle. They started pouring down the steep concrete steps of Stairway 13 at the Copland End, the traditional end for the home supporters in a local derby. Suddenly, with just thirty seconds left, a roar went up from the crowd: Colin Stein had scored an equaliser for Rangers. The flow of fans down the steps suddenly checked as they heard the roar, then somebody stumbled. The stream of fans building up behind fell over those lying in front, bodies starting to tumble over each other, just as the main body of fans started down the stairway following the final whistle. They piled on top of those already there, and the tumbling bodies turned into a cascade, the sheer weight of numbers bending the crush barriers and railings which were designed to resist just such an incident.

When the avalanche of people stopped, hundreds of fans had finished up in a huge pile at the bottom of the stairs, crushing to death those who ended up at the bottom. The uninjured and some of the 350 policemen at the stadium started to pull people out of the pile and give such first aid as was possible, but it took a long time for ambulances and medical teams to arrive. The match had finished at 4.46p.m., but the first 999 call was not made until 5.02. As ambulances from all over Glasgow converged on Ibrox, they found the streets teeming with the 80,000 spectators who had been at the match, most of whom had left without knowing what was happening on Stairway 13.

Nurses from local hospitals were among the first medically trained people to arrive, and they tried giving the kiss of life to many of the victims, but despite their efforts, sixty-six people died and 108 were seriously injured, Britain's worst football disaster to date.

At the time, unlike the English FA, Scottish clubs did not have to have their grounds certified by the Scottish FA, and many lacked the funds to invest in safety measures. Safety at British stadia was improved slowly, but it was always with the idea of retaining the traditional terracing rather than having all-seater grounds. The clubs were resistant, partly because of the cost and partly because it would mean changing the nature of the game for supporters, for whom the terracing with its history and atmosphere was all part of the attraction.

On Saturday 11 May 1985, Bradford City Football Club's Valley Parade ground was packed for its home game with Lincoln City. It was a great day for Bradford: they had just won the Third Division Championship and the trophy was to be presented before the match kicked off at 3p.m. It was a good-natured crowd, and when some fans threw a smoke bomb on to the pitch, they were quickly and quietly ushered away. There were 3500 people in the main stand, 2000 of them seated. At the time, there was great pressure from the football authorities to put high fencing in front of the stands to stop pitch invasions, but at Valley Parade, there was just a waist-high wall.

The match had been under way for thirty minutes when there was a long delay while one of the Lincoln players was carried off with a suspected broken leg. During the break, fans in the main stand saw smoke rising from underneath the seating; some thought it was another smoke bomb and reported it to the police. A policeman started searching for a fire extinguisher, but there were no fire-fighting facilities in the seventy-seven-year-old stand and the fire quickly caught hold among the debris which littered the ground under the seating. There was a stiff breeze blowing into the stand and suddenly the fire spread, fanned by the wind, and quickly reached the roof which was made of old timbers covered with asphalt. There was panic as the fire engulfed the stand, roaring up to the roof in a matter of minutes and scattering drips of hot tar and hunks of burning wood on to the people below. Many simply started scrambling over other people in their seats, either towards the back of the stand or to the front. At the back, they found the exits had been locked and the turnstiles would not let them out. Many then surged forwards again towards the front where a small wall separated the stand from the pitch. There were quite a number of elderly people in the stand who could not get over the wall, and the heat was so intense that many of them caught fire before they could get out, their clothes and hair simply starting to burn.

People were dying at the back of the stand, so policemen and fans from the other parts of the ground rushed forwards to help, and started pulling people over the wall while others went to the rear and smashed down the padlocked gates into the stand to let those trapped at the back escape; many people said later that they owed their lives to that quick thinking.

In the midst of the panic there were acts of great humanity and courage. David Hustler was trying to get out of the stand when he saw a woman in the seating area in a state of shock; she could barely move, so he helped her forward and over the wall. He had severe burns to his head, hands and legs, but when he saw a boy still in the stand with his clothes on fire, he climbed back over the wall to get him over too and managed to push him to safety before going over himself. Richard Gough had already escaped from the stand over the wall when he looked back and saw a woman with her hair on fire who could not get over the wall; he went back and dragged her over.

The police who had been there to control the match were among the first rescuers. PC Richard Ingham was on duty on the pitch when he saw a woman struggling just inside the perimeter wall, her clothes and hair on fire. He took an overcoat from a colleague and put it over his head, went into the stand and brought her back on to the pitch where he rolled her on the ground to extinguish the flames. Meanwhile, one of his colleagues, PC David Britton, was trying to help a man who was struggling to get over the wall with all his clothes alight. Once he was over, PC Britton started dousing the flames, but in the process, his own hair caught fire. PC Ingham saw what was going on and went to help, dragging the man further on to the pitch while PC Britton doused his own hair. At that point Ingham had to give up because the heat had completely exhausted him.

Chief Inspector Charles Mawson saw a man ablaze on the wall who could not get over, so he went in and pulled him to safety. Inspector Slocombe helped evacuate people over the wall until his tunic caught fire. Undeterred, he borrowed another officer's tunic and went back to rescue an old man caught on the wall. Had there been high fencing on the wall, people would have been trapped and the death toll would have been infinitely higher.

The fire service had been called at 3.46p.m. and arrived three minutes later, quickly putting in calls to nearby brigades to supply additional appliances. Eventually there were seventy-five firemen, ten pumps and twelve other vehicles on the scene, but they were unable to make much of an impression on the fire immediately, it was too intense.

Four ambulances were sent at 3.49 swiftly followed by two more, but once the scale of the disaster became apparent, fourteen ambulances were eventually called to the scene from as far away as Keighley and Halifax. Like Ibrox, the throng of people leaving the ground hampered the ambulances getting to it. When the crews got

Overleaf: The main stand at Valley Parade, Bradford City's football ground, ablaze from top to bottom on 11 May 1985.

133

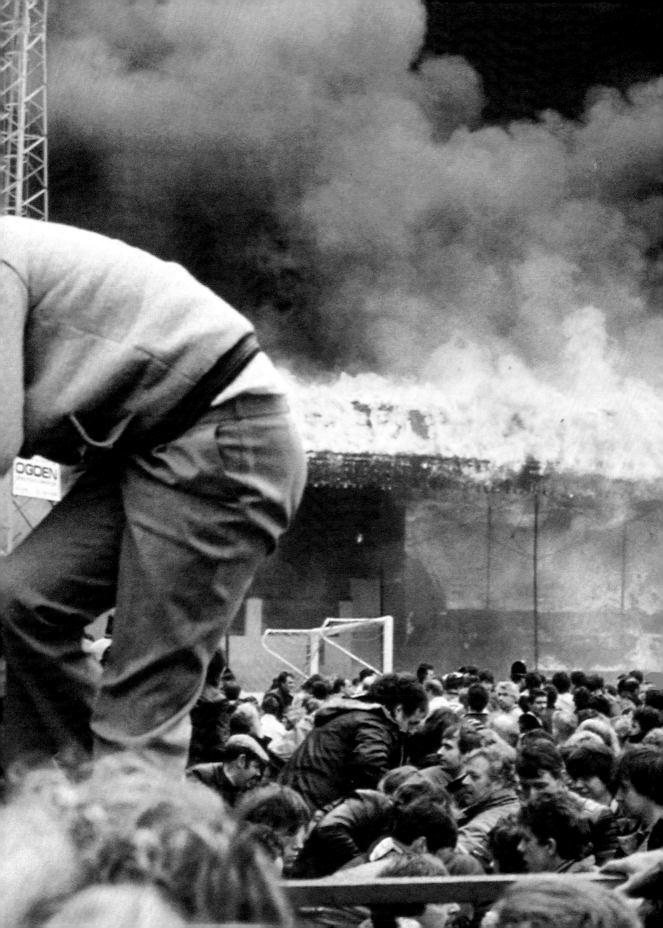

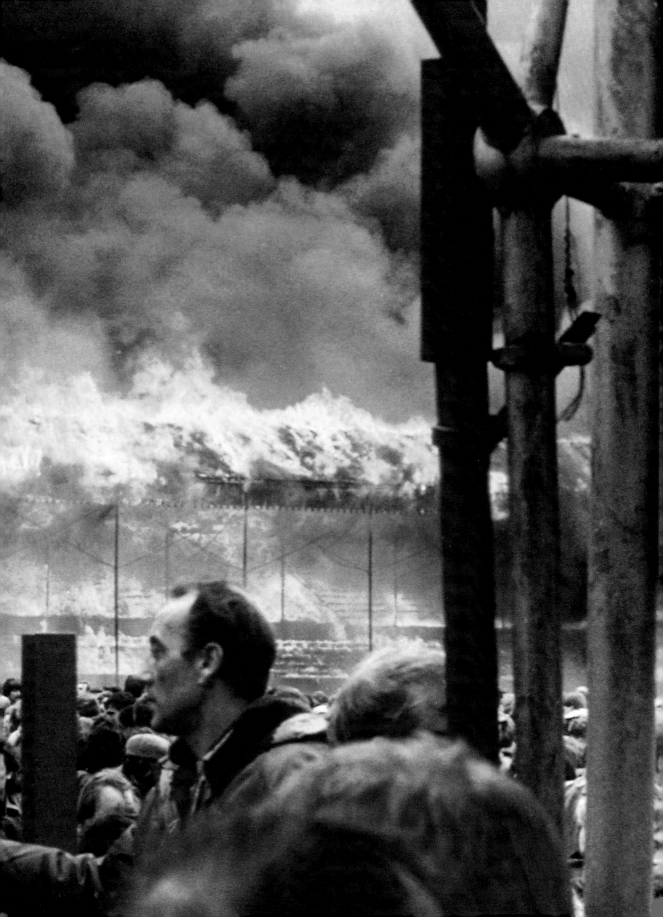

there, they found a great many injured people waiting in the road outside the ground – people with severe burns mainly to the scalp, hands, back and back of the legs. In the meantime, police cars and private cars were brought into service alongside the ambulances to ferry the first forty people to hospital.

At the Bradford Royal Infirmary, emergency procedures had been put into effect at 3.50p.m. and the casualty department told to prepare to receive a large number of burns cases. When they came, it was too much for one hospital. Around 200 admissions were made, but to treat them properly, a series of high-speed dashes by ambulance was arranged to take some patients to burns units at St Luke's Hospital in Bradford, to Pinderfields Hospital in Wakefield and to Batley General Hospital. Thirty people were kept in the BRI for surgery, and people were still coming into the hospital on Sunday suffering from the after-effects of smoke inhalation. Many of the burns victims had to have prolonged periods of treatment after the fire and many more suffered psychological traumas for a long time afterwards.

The fire fighters had the fire under control by early evening and it was officially pronounced out at 8.26p.m. The death toll was fifty-two. The cause was eventually put down to a lighted cigarette falling down between the floorboards of the stand and igniting the debris underneath. Six people won the Queen's Gallantry Medal for their bravery, among them David Hustler, Inspector Slocombe, PC Ingham, Chief Inspector Mawson and PC Britton.

Hooliganism played no part in the Bradford fire, but violent behaviour was a growing problem for the game as a whole. On the same day as the fire, Birmingham was playing Leeds at home. Just before half time, Birmingham scored a goal, Leeds fans invaded the field and a pitched battle started, first against the police, then between rival fans. Missiles of many kinds, from bricks and iron bars to bottles and coins, were used and inflicted many serious injuries, especially on the police. First aid cover was provided by the St John Ambulance who treated around 100 people before the game was restarted. More violence erupted after the game, putting over fifty people in hospital.

The same violent impulse infected international football too, particularly with British supporters. Greater mobility by air and sea meant that they could travel to the Continent for matches and sometimes that meant widespread brawling between fans in bars around the grounds before the match, and often simple vandalism on the trains and ferries to and from matches. Clubs always blamed small minorities of supporters – which was certainly true – but it was that minority which the non-footballing public saw as the unacceptable face of football and demanded change.

Two weeks after the Birmingham pitched battles and the Bradford disaster, on 29 May, the European Cup Final was being played between Liverpool FC and the Italian club, Juventus, at the Heysel stadium in Brussels, Belgium. Liverpool fans went on the rampage, charging the Italian and Belgian supporters who fled and were crushed against a safety wall. The wall gave way and forty-one died, many of them trampled to death, others crushed. Police and ambulance crews were called, and the fighting went on even as they were treating the wounded. The following day, Belgium banned British teams from competing in Belgium, then the day after that the Football Association banned all British teams from Europe. Two days later, UEFA banned British clubs from Europe 'indefinitely'.

It was the low point of British football in Europe. Clearly it would be a long time before British clubs would be allowed back into European competitions. To help them respond to the violence, the police set up special units to gather intelligence on the minority of troublemakers, and police officers from the home towns of clubs would swap information prior to a match between them, pre-empting trouble. But policing the front line between rival

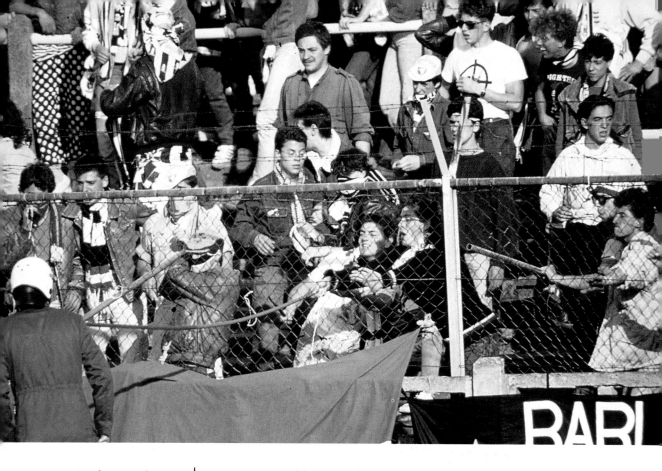

Low point for British football: Liverpool fans engaged in the violence on the terraces at the Heysel Stadium in Brussels which resulted in British teams being banned from European competition.

supporters and between football and the public was not the answer. To change, football would have to reform from within and give up some of its traditions, and all the police could do in the meantime was hold the front line. For their part, the clubs' contribution to holding the front line was to separate the rival fans at games by caging them in the terracing using thick wire fencing, making it impossible to invade the pitch or get at each other.

On Saturday 15 April 1989, Liverpool was playing in the semi-final of the FA Cup against Nottingham Forest at Sheffield Wednesday's Hillsborough ground, a quite modern stadium in a residential area of Sheffield. There were 800 police on duty to control the crowd and thirty volunteers from St John Ambulance with two of their ambulances, backed up by two more ambulances from the Sheffield City Ambulance Service.

Liverpool had by far the greater number of fans wanting to

attend and many of them arrived without tickets. They were also late because of traffic on the motorways and because of the routing which the police had prescribed for their coaches to keep them away from the Nottingham supporters. As the 3 o'clock kick-off time approached, there were long queues at the Leppings Lane entrance where around 4000 Liverpool fans were trying to get in to the West Stand. The crush of people steadily increased as ticket holders and those without tickets were processed through the entrances. As the kick-off approached, the crush was so great that even police horses trying to control the crowd were lifted off their feet. The senior police officer at the gate, Superintendent Roger Marshall, decided that there was a danger that they might push over the wall and it would be better to let them in whether they had tickets or not by opening a pair of wide gates, which were normally only opened at the end of a game to let people out.

The gates opened. Opposite them was a tunnel under the West Stand which led to the entrances to three sections of terraces which accommodated 10,000 standing spectators; above them there was

Hillsborough, Sheffield, 15 April 1989: Liverpool supporters caught in the crush which followed the surge of fans into the terracing in the West Stand are hauled up by fellow fans in the seating area above.

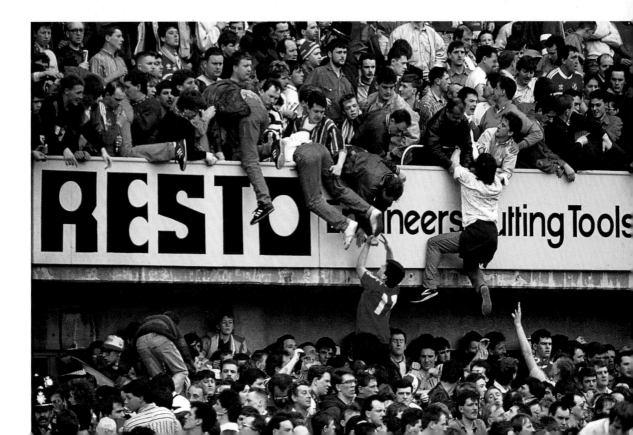

room for seated spectators. Along the whole front of the stand was an eight-foot-high wire-mesh fence to stop spectators invading the pitch. There were three sections, or pens, one in the centre, and two on either side with their own entrance on the end of the stand. The game was just starting when the gates opened, letting in thousands of fans who went straight for the central section, pouring into the tunnel and into the already tightly packed terrace beyond, immediately behind the Liverpool goal. Those inside were crushed up against the fence where many of them quickly had difficulty breathing. The fence was designed to keep people in and the top of it was bent inwards making it almost impossible to scale.

Elsewhere in the crowd, nobody seemed to realise what was going on. Some were aware of a disturbance in the terracing of the West Stand and at the Nottingham end of the ground, fans jeered and booed suspecting it was simply Liverpool fans engaged in some form of violent behaviour. The game went on as people were dying. It was a policeman on the pitch who realised their plight and he opened a small gate in the front of the fencing, but so tight was the crush that only a few people could make it out that way. A few of the more agile managed to escape over the top of the fence while others began to lift each other up to reach those in the seating area who could see the problem and started to pull them to safety.

Six minutes after the kick-off, a policeman ran out on to the pitch and told the referee to stop the game which he did, sending the teams back into the dressing rooms. Over the intercom, the Liverpool manager, Kenny Dalglish, asked people to cooperate with the police, then the Nottingham Forest manager, Brian Clough, followed suit.

The fire brigade was called at 3.14p.m. and arrived eight minutes later with rescue equipment and oxygen, but the firemen were unable to get help to where it was needed, in the tightly packed stand and the tunnel leading to it. Ambulances were delayed because the roads outside the Leppings Lane end were still milling with fans and the police were not able to clear a path. When the ambulances did arrive, some twenty minutes after the first spillage on to the pitch, they started ferrying the injured to the Royal Hallamshire and Northern General Hospitals.

Inside the stadium, Dr John Ashton, Professor of Medicine at Liverpool University, who was there to watch the match, made his way to the area behind the stand near the turnstiles where he arrived around twenty minutes after the game had been stopped. There was little he could do: there were no defibrillators – devices which supplied an electric shock to the patient's chest to restart the heart – nor was there any oxygen. Other doctors and nurses at the game tried to help, but they had no equipment either.

Peter Wells, the leader of the St John Ambulance Brigade team at the site, moved his band of young volunteers up to the fencing where people were being handed over the top, but there were still many people pressed up against it inside, dying. Wells tried to keep a young woman of around twenty alive by reaching through the mesh and trying to keep her mouth and airway open, but it was no use and she died. His wife, Kathy, was trying to resuscitate a boy of around ten on the pitch while his father looked on, then a doctor came by and told her to stop, that the boy was dead and she should try to save somebody else.

Behind the fences, those who fell down were crushed by others falling on top of them. One survivor described how he managed to get to the gate just as a boy in front of him stumbled and he fell on top of the boy as more people heaped on top of him, crushing the boy underneath as he fought for air. Friends were separated in the crush, fathers from sons and daughters. People saw their loved ones die, vomiting and turning blue before they did so. So strong was the force of the crush that the steel barriers in the terracing, designed to withstand 400lb per square inch to protect people on

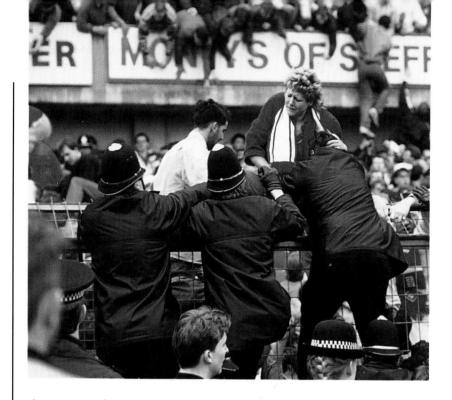

Police officers help Liverpool fans to climb over the fencing designed to keep fans off the pitch; instead, it trapped them in a terrifying crush of humanity which killed ninety-five people.

the terraces from being pushed over, were now bent over like pipe cleaners.

One man, Michael Murphy, was crushed inside the stand but he managed to lift many others up to the waiting hands in the seating area above. When he was exhausted, he was lifted up himself, then he went down to the pitch and gave mouth-to-mouth resuscitation to others. On the pitch, young men tore up advertising hoardings to carry their friends to the ambulances waiting outside.

It took a long time for the pressure to be relieved but eventually people did start to get out through the gate in the fencing in greater numbers where some collapsed and others tried to revive them with mouth-to-mouth resuscitation. Sheer pressure from inside burst the fencing in some places and firemen eventually managed to peel back part of the fence to allow more people to escape. Some were still alive; others were dead. Some bodies simply lay where they were.

From the three other stands, spectators who had come to watch a football game on a sunny spring afternoon suddenly found themselves gazing down on a pitch where a scene of chaos was unfolding: police; stewards; desperate fans running with bodies on makeshift stretchers; a lone ambulance parked in the Liverpool goal; desperate people trying to save others' lives by heart massage and the kiss of life. There was a cheer when one man seemed to revive, but it died away when it was clear he was dead. At home, relatives watched the scene on television.

There were no adequate medical facilities in the ground. The St John Ambulance volunteers worked hard, but they were not

A Liverpool supporter in the West Stand at Hillsborough, alone amid the debris following football's worst disaster.

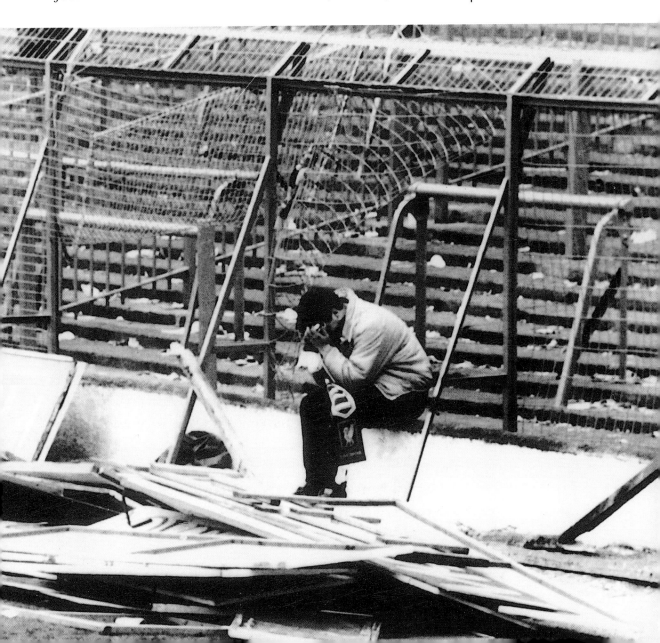

trained for an emergency on this scale, nor in the use of oxygen which would have saved lives – but there was no oxygen anyway.

Youngsters, both first-aiders and fans, showed how some people rise to the occasion. After the first surge, Ian Clarke, aged sixteen, was helping to try and drag unconscious spectators clear when he was buried under a pile of people during a second surge in the crush. He passed out under the pile of bodies but a policeman pulled him clear and he came round lying on the pitch. Once he was conscious again, he started giving mouth-to-mouth resuscitation to others lying on the pitch. Steven Holmes and Kevin Haymer, who had managed to get over the fence when the crush had first started, ripped off hoardings and made fourteen journeys back and forth to the ambulances carrying injured adults.

The scene behind the stand in the turnstile area was worse, bodies lying all the way down the steps to the terracing and around the turnstiles. People were carrying others to waiting ambulances outside in no particular order of priority. Dr John Ashton was trying to sort out priorities, differentiating between the dead, the dying and the seriously injured and deciding who should go to hospital first. It was 4.15 before the first casualty team arrived from a local hospital.

The Hillsborough gymnasium was turned into a temporary mortuary and it started filling up. The eventual death toll on the day was ninety-four, with another 400 people injured. On the Sunday, of the forty-eight people who were kept in the Northern General, fifteen were still in intensive care, all of them unconscious.

On the Sunday, Prime Minister Margaret Thatcher visited the survivors in hospital, as did the Prince and Princess of Wales on the Monday. In the early morning of the following day, one of the little boys whom they had visited died, bringing the total to ninety-five. It rose to ninety-six in 1992 when Tony Bland, who had been in a coma since the day of the disaster, died following a

High Court action which permitted his life support system to be switched off.

The recriminations were not long coming. The South Yorkshire Police took most of the blame though the Chief Constable of South Yorkshire, Peter Wright, defended his officers stoutly, determined not to have any of their actions pre-judged. But the view that the order to open the gate had caused the disaster was widely reported. The gate was opened with the best of intentions, but the action was tragically misguided. So was the policy of penning supporters in. Clubs with matches the following Saturday – big clubs such as Tottenham and Derby County – who had invested in fencing, started taking it down. At Anfield, Liverpool's home ground, there was no match. Liverpool went into mourning and the ground became a shrine for the week following the tragedy, the pitch strewn with millions of flowers as over two million people filed through the stadium to share their grief.

Blame for what had happened was laid at many doors, not least the police for opening the gates. The temperature of the debate was raised when the President of UEFA, Frenchman Georges Jacques, speaking of the Liverpool fans suggested that they had wanted to charge the stadium, that they had behaved like beasts. Two weeks later, fourteen Liverpool fans were each sentenced to three years' imprisonment in Belgium for their part in the Heysel Stadium disaster.

An inquiry into the Hillsborough disaster was set up, and Lord Justice Taylor published an interim report on 4 August, placing the blame firmly on the police for mishandling the arrangements at the game. Chief Superintendent David Duckenfield, who had been promoted from Chief Inspector only twenty-one days before the match, was accused of 'lying in the aftermath of the disaster'. Chief Constable Peter Wright offered his resignation, but it was not accepted. Of Superintendent Roger Marshall, who had ordered the gates to be opened, the report said that his 'capacity to take decisions [during the disaster] and give orders seemed to collapse'.

Violence did not cause the disaster at Hillsborough, but fear of violence and the measures designed to contain it greatly contributed to it. The wire-mesh pens and the police action, both measures designed to control the crowds and avoid trouble, created the circumstances that made the tragedy possible.

The disaster, once it happened, was on a scale which the emergency services were not able to respond to with the necessary speed. Clearly mistakes were made, but the Hillsborough disaster showed graphically that the heart of the problem was that changes over time in the numbers, mobility, rivalry and attitude of football supporters had changed the nature of the game dramatically; the modern game had outstripped the facilities at football grounds planned for a different age.

The real result was that the government, after yet another disaster, decided that the days of terracing were over for ever and that in future stadia would have to be all-seater; the national game would have to give up its traditions and change.

Chapter Six

TRAINS AND BOATS AND AEROPLANES

We live in an age of unprecedented mobility. From George Stephenson's *Rocket* to Concorde, some of the most spectacular and innovative uses of new technologies have been to find more and faster ways of travelling: steam trains, electric trains, diesel trains, underground trains, ocean liners, hovercraft, hydrofoils, catamarans, ro–ro ferries, airships, helicopters, jumbo jets, luxury coaches, forty-ton trucks and, above all, faster cars to drive on wider motorways, through longer tunnels under mountains and seas, over bridges across rivers and estuaries. From the outset though, that same quest for speed and mobility has produced some of the most spectacular man-made disasters and personal tragedies of the nineteenth and twentieth centuries, starting with the earliest mass transport system, the railway.

In 1879, a train set out over the Tay Bridge in Scotland during a severe storm, just as the bridge was swept away by fierce winds and seas. The train dropped into the water below and seventy people died, beyond the reach of any rescuers. Britain's worst ever train crash was in 1915 when 158 people were killed in a crash near Gretna Green. After the Second World War, there was a spate of fatal railway crashes. Between 1945 and 1952 there were fatalities

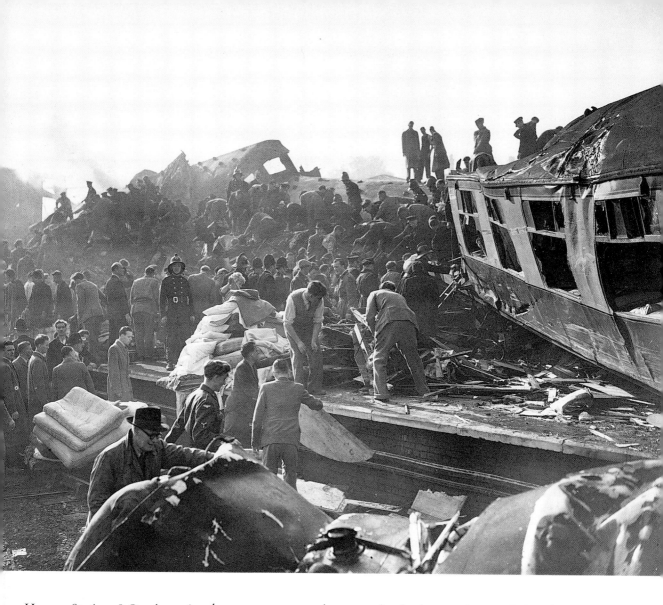

Harrow Station, 8 October 1952: firemen, servicemen, railway workers, policemen and passengers scramble through the wreckage in search of survivors of a crash in which three trains collided, killing 118 people.

almost every year, the worst by far happening on 8 October 1952 when a London-bound express train went through a danger signal outside Harrow station, smashing straight into the back of a commuter train standing in the station. The coaches of the two trains piled up on to the platform and the wreckage had hardly settled when, minutes later, the Liverpool-bound express came through Harrow at full speed in the opposite direction and ploughed into what was left of the first two trains. After many hours of work, the rescuers announced that the final death toll was 118.

South London, with its maze of commuter railway lines spreading out across southern England, has been the scene of a number of serious crashes. On 4 February 1957, ninety-two people were killed when two trains crashed in fog outside Lewisham, right underneath a bridge which then collapsed on top of the wrecked trains. On 5 November 1967, fifty-three people were killed and ninety injured at another south London junction, Hither Green.

In the 1980s, the signal system for the South-East Region was being extensively modernised. On Monday 12 December 1988, the 6.30a.m. fast train to London left Bournemouth for Waterloo with 468 people on board; the driver was John Rolls. At 7.18, a commuter train left Basingstoke, Hampshire, also bound for Waterloo with 906 people on board; the driver was Alexander McClymont. At 8.03a.m. an empty train left Waterloo for Haslemere.

At 8.13, Alexander McClymont, the driver of the Basingstoke train, saw a flickering signal as he approached Clapham Junction,

Spencer Park, Clapham, South London, 12 December 1988: ambulances and fire engines queue up alongside the railway tracks where three trains collided in the morning rush hour.

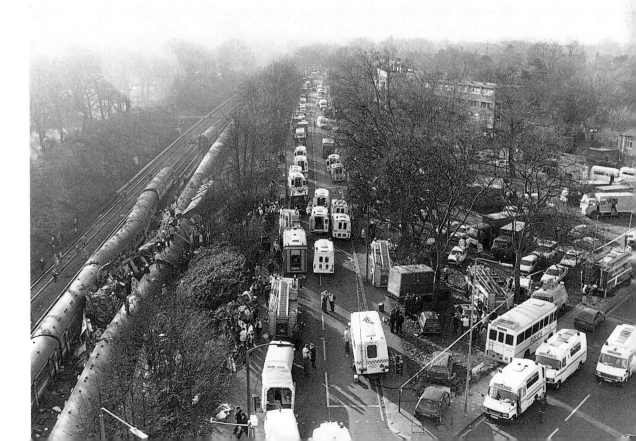

As firemen searched the wreckage, priority was given to finding those who were alive and giving them intravenous drips and painkilling drugs until they could be freed.

the busiest railway junction in Britain at the busiest time of day on the network. It was flickering from red, for 'stop', to amber, for 'prepare to stop', to green, for 'proceed'. He stopped at a track-side telephone to report it to the signal box. As he was speaking, the Bournemouth express, which had passed the signal, ploughed into the back of his stationary train with a huge crash which was heard throughout the immediate area. The express, its front a mangled mass of metal with gaping holes along the roofs and sides of the carriages, veered off into the path of the empty train from Waterloo which was on the next line, spilling passengers into its path. Some of those who had survived the initial crash were hit by the oncoming train. At 8.15 the guard on the empty train flagged down a fourth train which was coming down from Waterloo, averting an even greater disaster.

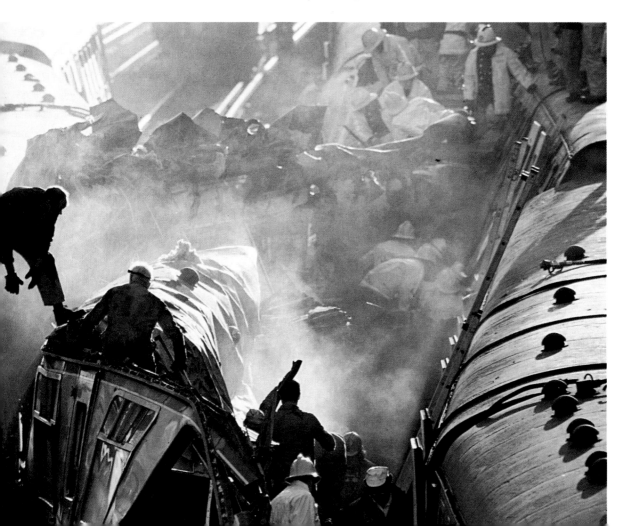

The two rear coaches of the Basingstoke train were thrown into the air, coming crashing down on their sides on the embankment. Passengers were hurled around inside their compartments, then trapped as the carriages disintegrated around them. In the express train, the impact forced the wheels and bogies up through the floor of the carriages, adding to the tangle of bodies, wood and steel.

The noise of the accident prompted many people to make 999 calls. A passing AA patrolman saw the accident and alerted the emergency services on his radio, then joined the rescue. The licensee of the Roundhouse pub nearby phoned the Battersea police station direct and the local police were there very quickly. Michael Matthews was passing in his car and saw the accident happen, dialled 999 on his car phone, then went down to help. Martin McCormack, a mechanic from Tooting, was on a bus going over Battersea Rise and saw it happen. He too went down the embankment and helped to pull people through broken windows.

On the embankment above the crash scene, three boys – Terry Stoppani, Joe Naylor and Peter Pantechi – were on the way to the Emmanuel Boys' School by bus. It was Terry's twelfth birthday. They scrambled over the fence and went down to the train. They were the first on the scene and what greeted them was gruesome; beside the track they saw the lower half of a body still dressed in jeans. Hundreds of uninjured and slightly injured people who had managed to get out of the trains were wandering around. The boys clambered on to the wrecked trains, got in through a broken window and started helping people out. One of their teachers, Mr John Wybrowe, scrambled over a six-foot-high wire fence on the other side of the track and crossed the electrified rails to join them. Another teacher, Mr George Cannon, was in the staff room when he heard the bang and went down to help before the emergency services arrived.

Separating the crash scene from the road was a ten-foot-high

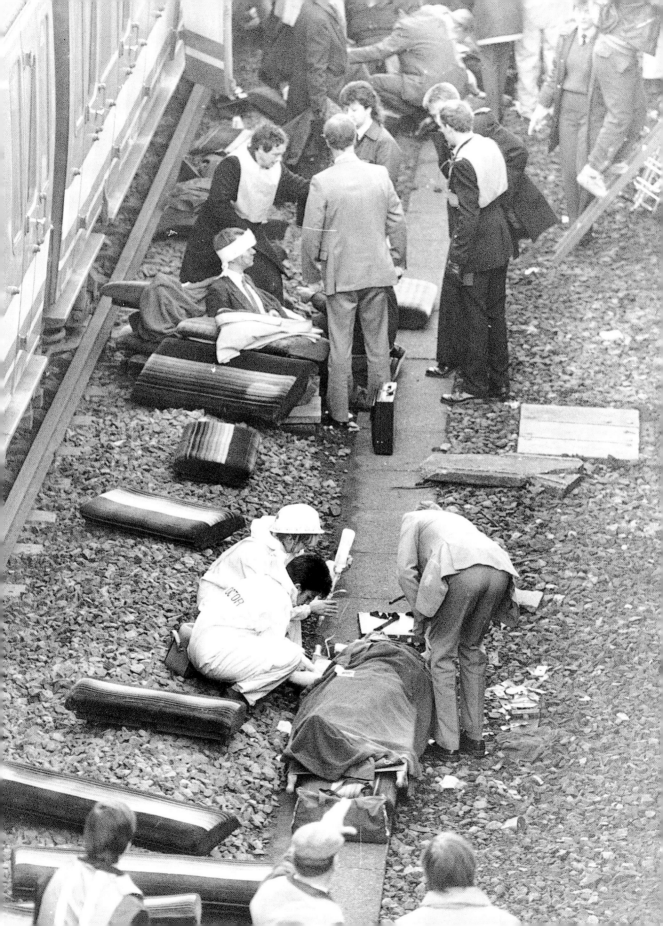

concrete wall which retained the bottom of a steep embankment covered in thick scrub. At the top of the embankment was a six-foot-high fence running along Spencer Park, a road which rapidly became a vehicle park for the emergency services.

Fire, police and ambulance stations were alerted at 8.17 and the major emergency plan put into operation immediately. The police were the first on scene and they started erecting traffic diversions and clearing a route for the ambulances and fire engines. The London Fire Brigade was next on the scene, only seconds after the police. In the second vehicle was Station Officer Mills who took charge on arrival, sending a message back to his control immediately asking for eight more appliances to be sent. Next he ordered his crews to use their short extension ladders to get down the concrete wall and help the walking wounded up, then went down to the scene himself to assess the situation. Even before he reached the bottom of the embankment, he radioed back for more fire engines and ambulances. Ten minutes after arriving, he sent out the message: 'This is a major incident.'

By this announcement, Mills ensured that all the emergency services and hospitals were alerted to the full nature of the accident. He then radioed for more fire brigade rescue tenders which carried the full range of cutting and lifting gear, and he ordered his men to take down the fence at the top of the embankment. When more senior fire brigade officers arrived to take control, Mills helped to carry up the first stretcher cases. The London Fire Brigade eventually sent fifteen fire appliances and 120 firemen to the crash.

The London Ambulance Service sent twenty-eight ambulances and eleven back-up coaches for the walking wounded. Forward control vehicles of all three services were parked close to each other in Spencer Park, establishing a control centre for the incident. Casualty wards at St George's Hospital in Tooting, which had only been opened the previous week, were made ready to receive large

Opposite: The swift arrival of skilled medical assistance at the Clapham rail crash saved many lives: two people trapped in the wreckage had to have limbs amputated on the spot; both survived.

numbers of casualties and a special resuscitation unit was established at the hospital. Two medical teams of doctors and nurses were sent from St George's to the scene. Two more medical teams were sent from St Stephen's in Fulham and one from St Thomas's in central London.

The Metropolitan Police helicopter landed nearby bringing doctors who belonged to a charity called BASICS, British Association for Immediate Care, and who specialised in working in disasters. At the crash scene, after an initial quietness, there was screaming from the wreckage.

At 8.21a.m., the first ambulances arrived and the scene which greeted them was one of carnage: hundreds of survivors, many of them in a state of shock, were struggling to climb up the embankment. Having set up their ladders, the firemen then used shovels to cut steps down the embankment, making it easier for survivors to get up and rescue services to get down.

There were bodies on the side of the tracks, but the medical teams which arrived concentrated on those who were still alive and trapped in the wreckage. They were equipped with saline drips, pain-killing drugs and blood for transfusions which they were able to administer on site. They had large quantities of a fluid called Haemaccel, used in the drips to stabilise patients, and Entonox, a gas used to kill pain. They also needed more blankets, stretchers and oxygen. When drugs and other medical supplies ran short, the police helicopter was used to collect them and fly them in because the roads were too congested.

Ambulance, police and fire crews shepherded the slightly injured up the embankment, and while ambulances started ferrying the badly injured to hospital, those who did not need urgent attention were taken to the Emmanuel School where the headmaster, Peter Thompson, organised his pupils into teams to help them, bring them tea and give first aid. The Roundhouse pub and other business premises were also opened up to shelter the walking wounded and let them use the telephones to tell their families and workplaces.

Television and radio carried reports of the crash all morning and one of the benefits of the publicity was to bring blood donors out in hundreds; within hours, there was a queue outside St George's Hospital waiting to give blood.

Once most of the injured had been taken up the embankment, the emergency services concentrated on searching the wreckage. Those who were trapped had to be cut out, or access to them provided by cutting passages through the destruction. This was done by firemen and there was all-round praise for the way they speedily got on with the job. Many of the injuries were fractures and crushed bones as bodies were trapped by huge pieces of railway engineering. Five seriously injured people trapped in the wreckage were stuck for several hours; two had to have limbs amputated on the spot.

Mr Paul Calvert was the leader of one of the medical teams which went into the wreckage; he was also the medical incident officer on site. He treated one woman who was still conscious whose hand was practically severed while also suffering from severe internal injuries to her spleen and liver, a fractured elbow, a thigh injury and a broken arm. Another man was pinned to the ground by a large piece of metal across his pelvis and his legs; he also had severe internal injuries. He was given strong pain-killing drugs and a saline drip as firemen, doctors and nurses treated him and released him together. He was the last living casualty to be released at 12.15p.m., four hours after the crash.

At 1 o'clock St George's Hospital announced that it had received 123 casualties of which forty-two had been detained. Prioritising those in need of the most immediate treatment was a crucial part of the casualty admissions process: in the resuscitation unit, five teams of doctors and nurses had the job of deciding who should go straight through to surgery and who could wait. Nine emergency operations were carried out, during which one patient died on the operating table despite strenuous efforts to save him. Sixty-nine people were seriously injured and 415 had minor injuries. What saved many people was medical teams getting to the spot quickly with enough supplies to keep them alive and get them to hospital in a condition which made successful operations possible.

At 5 o'clock, the London Fire Brigade announced that all the bodies had been removed from the wreckage, but the final death toll took some time to establish because of the number of dismembered bodies. It eventually reached thirty-three, with two more people dying later from their injuries; all of them had been in the first two carriages of the Bournemouth train. The cause of the disaster was faulty wiring installed by a technician engaged in the modernisation of the signalling system.

There was universal praise for the speed and efficiency of the emergency services and for members of the public who helped, and that effectiveness contributed hugely to saving life. Speed in getting medical help to the victims of a crash, stabilising them and getting them to hospital as quickly as possible was the key.

The idea of bringing speedy medical attention to the patient, then evacuating them to the best hospital for the type of treatment they need was behind the establishment of the Helicopter Emergency Medical Service based at the London Hospital in August 1990.

On 8 January 1991, a tightly packed commuter train crashed into the buffers at Cannon Street station a couple of miles from the London Hospital. A great many people were trapped in the wreckage. Fire rescue services were on the scene very quickly and started freeing people, but so was the HEMS helicopter which landed on the rails, very near the platform. Doctors from the London, Bart's

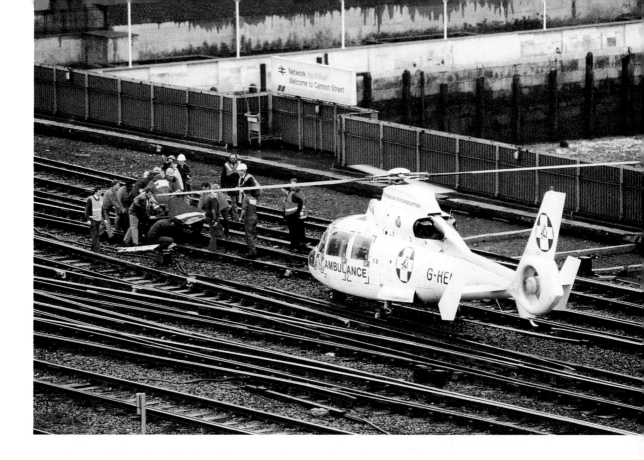

and Guy's assessed the casualties on site and those in need of urgent attention went by air to the London, flown directly to the roof of the hospital over the congested streets. Ambulances were on the scene within six minutes and the first casualties were in hospital within thirty-one minutes of the crash. The London Hospital took twenty-two casualties, St Bartholomew's took 107, and Guys 130, of whom thirty-one in total were kept in overnight; one passenger died.

The railways created the commuter and today millions of people depend on trains to transport them from home to work, but in London the first Underground railway was opened in 1863 to link the mainline stations. For most of its 130-year history, the London Underground has had an excellent safety record. The worst accidents have all been in this century and the numbers killed in each

Speed of evacuation has become the essence in crash medicine and rescue. When a crowded commuter train crashed into the buffers at Cannon Street station on 8 January 1991, the HEMS helicopter, with Accident and Emergency consultant surgeon Mr Alastair Wilson on board, landed two minutes after it was alerted, within yards of the injured.

The scene at Moorgate Underground station on 28 February 1975 when a train crashed into a dead-end tunnel: the fight to free trapped passengers went on for eighteen hours before everybody was accounted for. Around 500 people took part in the rescue.

never reached double figures: five people died in a collision on the Metropolitan Line in 1924; six people died in a collision on the District Line in 1938; three people were killed in a collision at Northwood in 1945; and three people died when two trains crashed at Stratford in 1953.

On 28 February 1975, that record was abruptly changed at Moorgate station in the City when the 8.37a.m. from Drayton Park was just approaching the end of its journey. The train was not packed, some carriages were about two-thirds full. The driver was Leslie Newson, aged fifty-six and in the rear carriage was the guard, Bob Harris, aged eighteen. As they approached the station, the guard and the passengers felt the train speed up a little instead of slowing down, followed by an almighty crash. Moorgate is a dead end with around 250 feet of tunnel beyond the platform

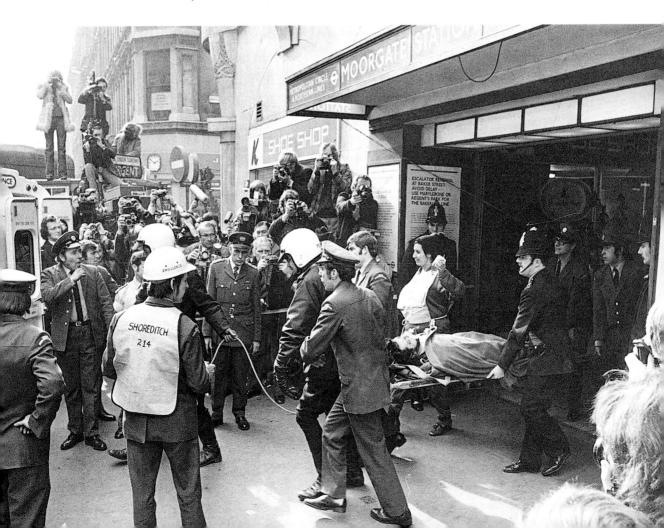

finishing with a sand trap then a wall. As the front carriage hit the wall, the first fifteen feet of it were compressed into no more than about two feet, such was the impact, and the whole carriage was reduced to about fifteen feet. Leslie Newson was killed instantly. The second carriage forced its way under the first and the third carriage forced its way on top of the second, leaving all three compressed into the cul-de-sac tunnel, mangling passengers and carriages together with no room to move around them. The impact of the crash released soot from the tunnel which filled the air clogging lungs and blackening faces.

The passengers in the last three carriages were not too badly injured, most were badly shaken but some were able to climb out of the broken windows and stagger on to the platform, which was in total darkness as the power had been cut. Many were still trapped in the wreckage and many of them were already dead. Bob Harris came forward from his position in the last carriage with a torch and shone it into the entrance to the tunnel where he could see bodies in the wreckage; a nurse was trying to free one woman who was trapped by twisted metal pressing down on her chest. People were shouting for help and screaming in pain, but there was little anybody could do.

Ambulances and fire engines were quickly on the scene at road level and ambulance staff and firemen started down, with portable lighting and oxy-acetylene cutting gear. They smashed windows to get into the carriages in the tunnel and brought out some of the walking wounded. People arriving at the surface were blackened by the smoke, soot and dust.

The rescuers were soon joined by doctors and nurses from all over London, including Bart's, who came to help when they heard about the crash on the radio. A steady stream of casualties were soon being carried up the two escalators. By mid-morning, seventy-eight badly injured people had been taken to St Bartholomew's

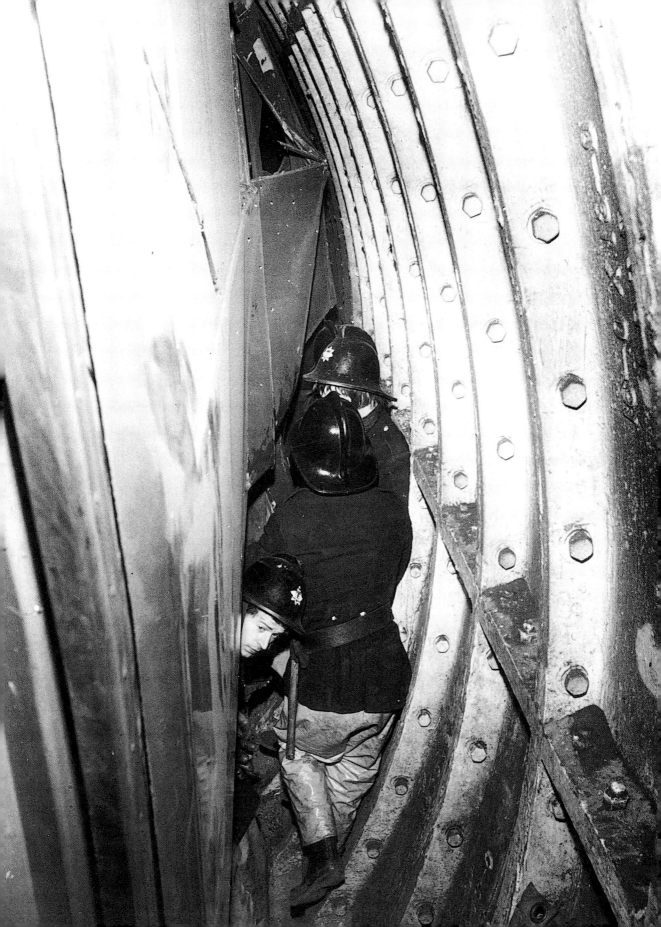

and the London Hospital, leaving the most difficult cases still trapped.

From the ticket barrier the sound of hammers and cutting gear went on all morning. The atmosphere on platform 9 was quiet, but it also became stiflingly hot. There was little or no ventilation and firemen were using oxy-acetylene torches to cut the metal. The rescuers entered the wreckage through the rear door of the third coach, which was pitched up at an angle of 45 degrees, then crawled through the wreckage using hydraulic jacks to open up gaps in the twisted metal. This way they created tiny passages for other rescuers and medical teams to crawl through, without bringing any of the wreckage down on the survivors or the rescuers. The men stripped to the waist in temperatures which reached 120 degrees Fahrenheit and after a while they could only work for twenty minutes at a time before coming up for a breather and a drink.

Opposite: Working conditions for the firemen were not only very cramped, the atmosphere was also stiflingly hot.

Below: Twenty minutes in the tunnel was all that doctors would permit the rescue workers, but despite the order, many firemen worked longer shifts in their keenness to save lives.

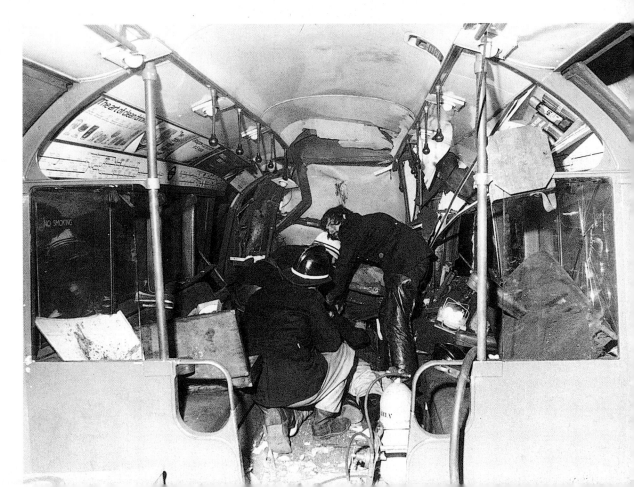

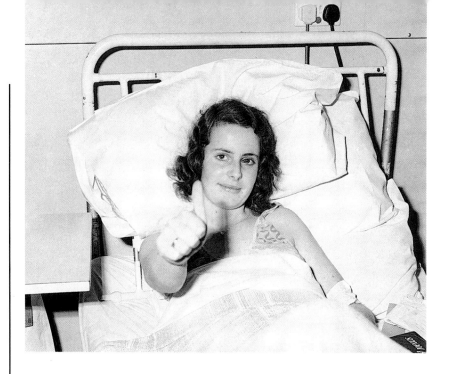

WPC Margaret Liles, aged nineteen, in hospital after being rescued by having her left foot amputated in order to free her and a fellow passenger.

The street above was cordoned off by police. Some 500 members of the emergency services were involved as a whole, with 100 people working directly in the tunnel at any one time. One of the greatest demands of the rescuers was drink, and to meet it the Salvation Army set up a tea caravan on the corner of Finsbury Circus. People wanted to help and Londoners responded in any way they could: a blood donor centre was set up in London Wall and within hours 800 people were queuing to give blood; taxi drivers refused fares for anybody going to help or give blood.

Only four or five rescuers could work inside the wreckage at any one time so progress was slow, but by afternoon, they were in contact with a nineteen-year-old policewoman, Margaret Liles, stationed at Bishopsgate station, who was trapped in the first carriage alongside a Stock Exchange broker, Jeff Benton, aged twenty-seven. There were six dead bodies close by. Margaret Liles was very lucid, cheery even, and she encouraged the rescuers to get out those more severely injured than herself even though her legs were buckled up underneath her. She was trapped by her left foot which was stuck underneath one of the huge bogies which had come up through the floor, and in order for the rescuers to get to Mr Benton, they had to get her out first and they could not get her out because of her trapped foot. They were the last two left alive.

The fire brigade was experimenting with a communications system called Figaro, which provided radio communications in just such disasters, and the rescuers managed to pass Margaret Liles a set which she was able to use. They also asked if she would like a WPC to come and sit with her, but she said she would prefer a male officer. Over the Figaro radio, she also chatted with her mother who had arrived in mid-afternoon and had been waiting on the surface in a police car for news of her daughter.

Jeff Benton was very badly injured and the only way to get them both out was to amputate Margaret Liles' foot on the spot; she agreed to sacrifice her foot to get Jeff Benton out. The operation was carried out by Mr Ashley Brown, a surgeon from Bart's. At 8.40p.m., after twelve hours ten minutes, she was brought out and reunited with her mother.

Then the rescuers freed Jeff Benton and brought him out too. He managed a cheery wave to the crowds above when he came out, but sadly he died a month after the accident. He was the last person brought out alive, but the teams worked on through the night to free the dead. On the surface, relatives waited in hope rather than expectation. By Monday they had brought out twenty-six bodies. When the rescuers reached the front of the wreck, they found Leslie Newson's body still in his cab. The final death toll was thirty-five.

Amid the tragedy of the Underground's worst crash, there was also the joy of having survived it. Margaret Liles, the heroine of the incident, was interviewed by press and television surrounded by mountains of flowers and cards after a second operation which removed her leg below the knee.

* * *

Blues and Twos

The top of the wooden-slatted escalators at King's Cross where the fire was started, probably by a lighted cigarette, before spreading to the booking hall where most of the dead were found.

Just two stops west of Moorgate on the Underground is King's Cross, the busiest station in London and one of the busiest in Europe. It is a huge junction in the system, bringing together the Metropolitan, Circle, Northern, Piccadilly and Victoria Lines, right under the British Rail station. The booking hall is served by two sets of escalators, both of the pre-war design using wooden-slatted steps. To the right are the escalators to the Victoria Line and to the left is the one serving the Piccadilly and Northern Lines.

The evening rush hour on Wednesday 18 November 1987 was drawing to a close but the station was still very busy at 7 o'clock. At 7.15, a member of the Underground staff had extinguished a small fire at the bottom of the Victoria Line escalator using a fire extinguisher and without calling the London Fire Brigade. Shortly afterwards, around 7.25, a fire started in grease and other detritus

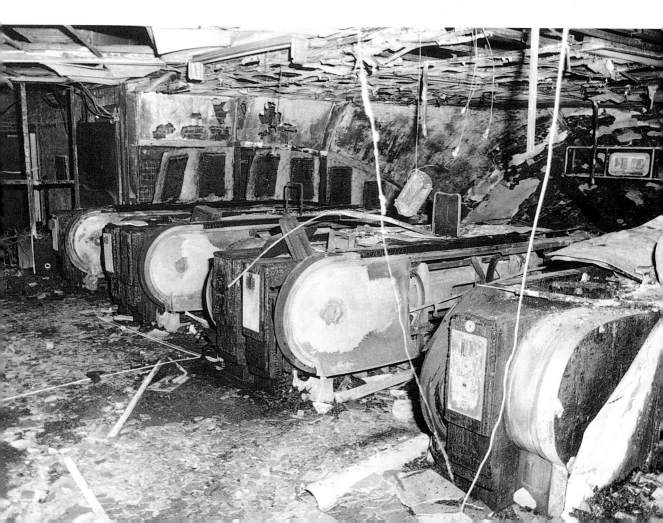

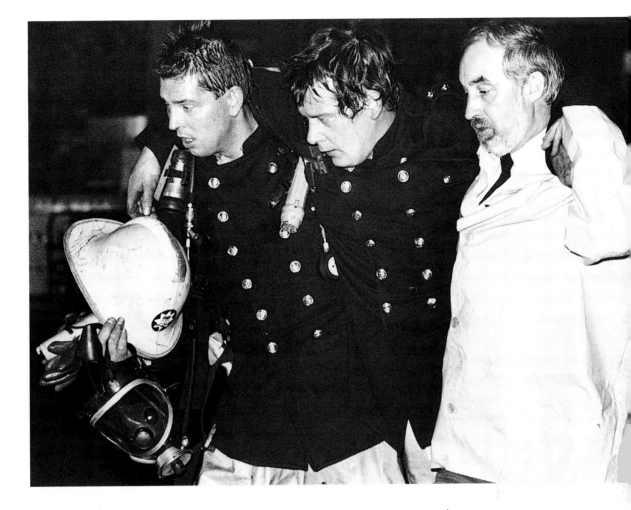

under the Piccadilly Line escalator, probably set off by a lighted cigarette which had been discarded on the escalator.

The fire was spread by the moving escalator and when Police Constables Kenneth Kerby, Steven Hanson and David Bebbington were called to the scene, they decided that the station should be closed. PC Bebbington dialled 999, reporting the fire and suggesting that trains should be instructed to go straight through the station.

The London Fire Brigade was summoned at 7.34p.m. and the first appliance arrived at 7.42. Station Officer Colin Townsley and

Firemen suffering from the effects of working in the booking hall area of King's Cross where they were trying to rescue people.

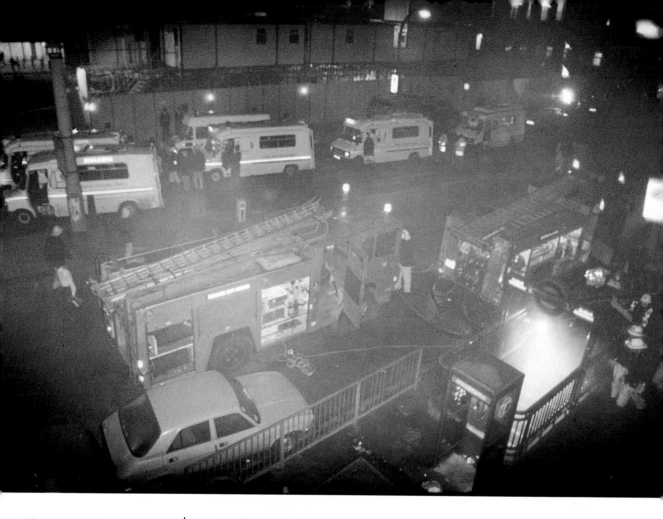

The scene outside King's Cross Underground station on 18 November 1987 as the emergency services gathered to tackle the fire which killed thirty-one people.

Sub-Officer Bell went into the booking hall from where they could see the fire burning about halfway up the up escalator. Bell went down the escalator to warn passengers not to use the up escalator while Townsley made a detailed inspection of the fire, then went back to the booking hall where he ordered firemen with breathing apparatus and a water jet to the fire. He also instructed Leading Fireman Flanagan to radio for four more pumps to attend the scene.

There were around 200 passengers waiting at the bottom of the Piccadilly Line escalator, and flames had reached the roof of the escalator shaft, but PC Hanson believed they had the situation under control. Suddenly there was a fierce explosion which many people who heard it described as a huge 'whoosh'. It sent out a

166

shock wave and it blew people off their feet. It was followed by a rolling sheet of flame from floor to ceiling across the whole of the booking hall and down the Victoria Line escalator shaft. It was subsequently described as a 'flashover', and the most likely explanation was that there had been a build-up of combustible gases in the roof space which were ignited by the fire on the escalator.

The flashover occurred at 7.45, just as the firemen detailed by Colin Townsley to fight the fire on the escalator were entering the booking hall. They were engulfed in it as it swept across the top of the hall. The heat was intense; it set clothes and hair alight and burnt skin without the flames even touching it. Richard Bates, a journalist on the *Guardian*, was on the up escalator from the Victoria Line when the flashover occurred. It burned his exposed skin and set his clothes on fire.

The flashover had stopped communications between those below and at the top. Bell, who was below and unaware of the flashover, was stopping people from going up the escalators and urging them to get back on the trains, believing that the fire would be tackled by men with breathing apparatus from the top. When he went back he saw that the fire was much worse and started to try to use the fire equipment available to fight it. Fighting the fire from below might have made it worse for the people above, but on seeing it was worse anyway, he started fighting it with the aid of PC Bebbington. They found a fire hose and went up the escalator bringing as much water to bear on it as possible. Three times they attacked the fire, but each time they did, it took hold again. They ripped off the side panels to the escalator to find the source of the fire underneath and attacked it with the hose again.

Meanwhile, confusion was setting in. Passengers on the Piccadilly Line platform could not get on to the trains since they were running straight through the station. The Victoria Line escalators ended up in the same booking hall, so many of them were directed away from the Piccadilly Line escalator to the Victoria Line exit, but when they did so, they went straight into the fire which may have led to some of them dying. The problem was that nobody on the platforms below knew about the fire in the booking hall. Station Officer Peter Osborne was in the booking hall as the flashover occurred. He was standing at the top of the Victoria Line escalator shouting to people to go back down because of the situation in the booking hall. Near the top of the escalator he saw a man with his clothes on fire, crouching down to avoid the smoke, then jumping over to the down side; it was Richard Bates. Osborne went down to the bottom and put out the fire on his clothes with an extinguisher, then had him evacuated by two policemen.

Outside, the firemen had lost contact with their officers, believing them to be dead. Using their own initiative, Firemen Moulton, Button and Flanagan tried to enter the booking hall to rescue people using breathing apparatus but were beaten back by the heat. Next Moulton went back with two other firemen playing their hoses on to his back to try and reduce the temperature. Inside, he found Colin Townsley's body close to the steps leading up to the St Pancras Road entrance, and close by was the body of a woman whom he had been trying to help escape when they were both overcome by the heat of the flashover.

At 7.49p.m. Assistant Divisional Officer Shore from Euston fire station arrived and found that none of his own officers was there to brief him, nor any Underground staff who could explain the labyrinth of passages at King's Cross. He ordered more fire pumps and four ambulances to attend. Once he realised that he had lost his senior officers, he ordered yet more pumps, if only because he knew that they would come with other senior officers who could help organise the fire fighting. Eventually there were thirty pumps and 200 firemen at the scene, and by 8.15p.m. liaison between fire, ambulance, police and Underground staff on

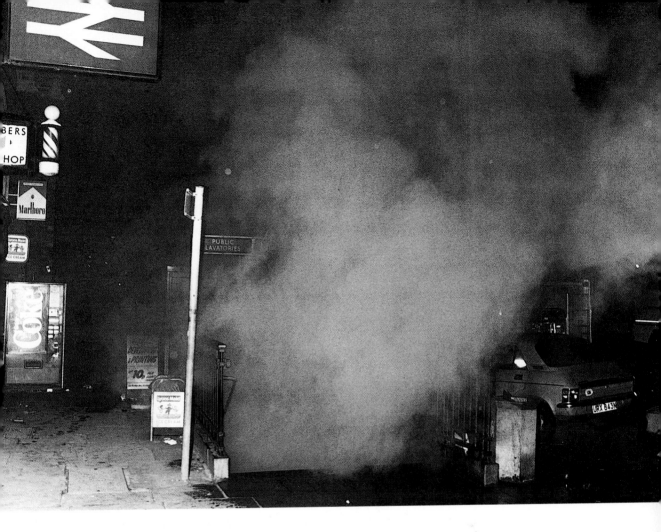

the surface was established, and though the fire was not out the situation was coming under control.

In the meantime, at 8.09 the ambulance service had declared the fire a major incident, putting local hospitals on alert to receive large numbers of casualties and call in extra staff. They started arriving at St Bartholomew's and University College Hospital shortly afterwards and surgeons were shocked at the severity of the burns caused by the flashover. By midnight, University College was unable to accept any more casualties.

One of the main problems was the complicated geography of the station. There was no map of the tunnels available; there were two in the ticket area, but it was engulfed in flames and smoke. At 9.48

Within minutes of the arrival of the fire brigade, a lethal mixture of gases which had built up in the ceiling space of the station booking hall exploded, causing most of the casualties.

169

the Fire Brigade announced that it had the 'fire surrounded' and by 1.42a.m. it was out. Thirty-one people died in the fire, many of them found at the top of the escalators where the flashover occurred and in the exits from the booking hall as they tried to escape.

The direct cause of the fire was a lighted cigarette or match falling on to rubbish which had accumulated underneath the escalator; the real cause was complacency. In his inquiry, which was published in November 1988, Mr Desmond Fennel QC made 157 separate recommendations about safety on the Underground and his comments about the approach to safety of the Chairman, Sir Keith Bright, led the latter to resign. Most damningly, the report pointed out that there had been many warnings long before the disaster about the danger of allowing rubbish to accumulate under the escalators.

Just as the railways created the commuter, so the car ferry began popularising the idea of touring holidays abroad, in Ireland and on the continent. On 31 January 1953, the British Rail car ferry *Princess Victoria* sailed out of Stranraer for Larne in Northern Ireland, and into mountainous seas. The guillotine car deck doors in the stern had not been closed properly and a large wave hit them, bursting them open and allowing water to pour into the car deck, sweeping cars and cargo to starboard. She soon developed a list to starboard and passengers were told to abandon ship. The radio operator, David Broadfoot, sent out an SOS message, but he only had a ship-to-shore radio, there was no open emergency channel which could be received by all ships in the area. The Master tried to make for Loch Ryan, but was unable to do so because of the weather. Broadfoot continued to send out radio messages trying to guide ships to their position. The order to abandon ship was given when the ship was over on her side, but

Broadfoot stayed at his radio as the passengers prepared to go.

By the time the first rescue ship arrived, the destroyer HMS *Rothesay*, she had drifted away from her reported position in the stormy weather and was within sight of the Irish coast. The passengers had plenty of time to put on their life jackets but many of them had to jump into the sea since a number of the lifeboats could not be lowered because of the list to starboard. There were forty-four survivors, but 128 were drowned, including the Master, Captain James Ferguson, and David Broadfoot who was posthumously awarded the George Cross for staying at his post when he might have escaped and survived.

The popularity of foreign holidays by car grew throughout the 1950s and 1960s, leading to the development of bigger, more efficient car ferries with huge doors at each end so that cars and lorries could drive on through one end of the ship and off through the other – roll on–roll off (ro–ro) ferries as they became known. Ro–ro ferries are perfectly designed for their task, with huge decks which can be loaded with cars quickly, but as ships they are lethal. If water gets inside the vehicle decks – even a small amount sloshing about on the wide, open decks with no bulkheads in between – it can destabilise the ships which are also very tall. If the vehicles on the deck then move they can capsize very quickly.

In 1982, five people died when two such ferries collided and one sank quickly. In the same year, another six people died – four crew and two passengers – when a Townsend Thorensen ferry, the *European Gateway*, was hit amidships and rolled over very quickly, fortunately in shallow water otherwise the death toll would undoubtedly have been much higher.

On Friday 6 March 1987, the evening sailing of Townsend Thorensen's *Herald of Free Enterprise* from the Belgian port of Zeebrugge to Dover scheduled for 7p.m. was delayed. It was her second round trip of the day, and she was loaded with around 600 passengers, most of them British, many of them Army families returning to Britain from service in Germany. There were eighty crew members, eighty-one cars and forty-seven lorries. The 7951-ton ro–ro ferry had been built in 1980 for the Dover–Calais route. At Calais there were two ramps for unloading, one for each of two decks, but at Zeebrugge there was only one and for loading, water was pumped into ballast tanks at the bow of the ship, tilting it slightly nose down so that both decks could be loaded from the single ramp.

Twenty minutes behind schedule the *Herald of Free Enterprise* sailed. The weather was very cold, with an east wind, but the sea was calm as she headed out into the harbour. Her bow doors were open, a practice which had sometimes been used on ro–ros to clear exhaust fumes from the car decks. As she accelerated to around fifteen knots, the combined effect of the slight nose-down attitude of the ship and sitting down lower in the water as she gained speed increased the bow wave, allowing water up over the forward ramp and on to the car deck.

She passed the outer mole of the harbour at 7.24p.m. Just outside the harbour, she tilted to port, righted again briefly, then tilted over again through 90 degrees to lie on her side, three-quarters of her under the water, her port side lying on a sand bank, her starboard side still above water. No alarm had been raised, it all happened too quickly. Evacuation procedures allowed for thirty minutes to get people off. It all happened in four minutes and if it had not been for the sand bank, almost certainly she would have turned right over.

There was no time to send a Mayday signal. The bridge was forty feet wide and as the ship turned over, so it became a vertical shaft. As the ship rolled Captain David Lewry and all those with him on the bridge tumbled down, finishing up at the bottom with the captain seriously injured. The suddenness caught passengers and crew completely unawares, and throughout the rest of the ship there was no question of a policy of women and children first – crew members helped people as they came along. It was so sudden that people sitting at tables in the restaurant and bar were thrown out of their seats and fell against the walls, breaking bones and being separated from one another. There was understandable panic as shelves full of drink, bottles, books, brochures, duty-free goods and glasses came crashing down. Against that was the sound of the sea water rushing into the ship. The restaurant quickly filled with water, the lights went out and people scrambled over each other in the darkness trying to reach safety.

People were screaming, trying to swim in rooms on their sides partially filled with water, with oil, life jackets with their fluorescent strips glowing in the darkness, personal belongings and, very soon, dead bodies, all around them. The water was bitterly cold. People struggled to use tables which were bolted to the floor as stepping stones. Emergency lighting came on but it was very dim and did not last long. What light there was came from what had been six-foot-square windows, but which were now skylights, letting in a weak light; they were what people made for.

The problem was that in making for safety, suddenly the internal layout of the ship presented great danger. What had been a corridor could now be a sheer drop; doors in what were walls now became trap doors in the floor as crew and passengers tried to find their way up to the starboard side, where rescue services were gathering.

Outside the rescue services had been alerted and they reacted swiftly. On the quayside, ambulances drew up waiting for the first casualties and the Belgian authorities put hospitals on alert. Tugs from the Dutch firm Smit came alongside as did helicopters from the Belgian and Dutch Navies. RAF Sea Kings were sent from RAF Culdrose with divers and thermal imaging cameras which could detect the living. Among the first divers to get to the wreck were

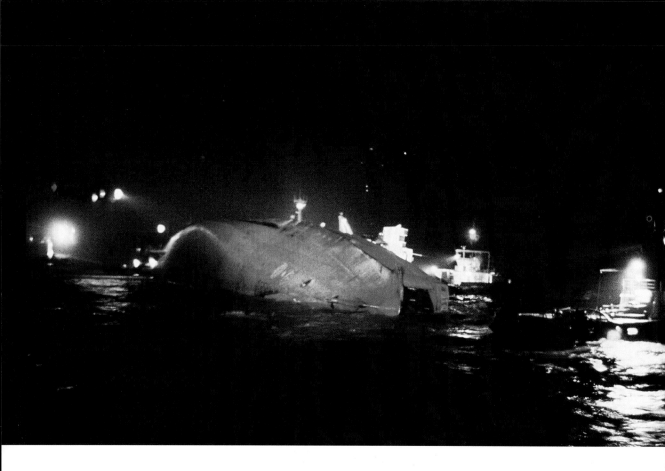

On her side, the *Herald of Free Enterprise* lies in darkness just outside Zeebrugge harbour surrounded by tugs and rescue craft. The first forty survivors were taken off by the dredger, *Sanderus*, after its master, Robert Heinemann had seen the car ferry turn over from around a mile away. He sent out the Mayday signal which alerted the authorities on shore to the emergency.

three British sailors from the minesweeper, HMS *Hurworth*, which was in Ostende, seventeen miles from Zeebrugge. Only one of them, nineteen-year-old Able Seaman Eamon Fullen, was on board when news came through to the ship about what had happened, but he collected the ship's diving gear, hijacked a car from a doctor, rounded up the other divers from shore leave and took a taxi to Zeebrugge.

As dusk gathered, helicopters brought searchlights which they shone down on the hull. When rescuers landed on the side of the ship, they could see people under the windows; it was the only way out, so they started smashing them.

There were hundreds of individual stories. An eight-year-old boy, Martin Hartley, described after he was rescued how people had scrambled over each other in their bids for safety, and how he and his father at one time were both knocked down and trodden on. Martin survived, but his parents and grandparents died. A soldier, Stan Mason, was returning from Germany with his wife and baby. He managed to keep hold of his baby daughter Kerry by gripping her clothes in his teeth while searching for his wife, whom he failed to find. Susan Hames and her German boyfriend were in the lounge when it happened. As the ship turned over, she grabbed the door and hung on to it as the water rushed in underneath her. She became separated from her boyfriend, but rose with the water and eventually found a ledge in the superstructure which she stayed on, removing her pullover and shoes. She could hear others around her but could see nothing. After half an hour, rescuers on the outside smashed through a window near her and let down a rope ladder and she climbed out.

Assistant Purser Stephen Homewood managed to find his way through the labyrinth to join a group of soldiers who had congregated in a stairwell near one of the exits which was open above them. They managed to get a routine going, making steps with

Rescuers working on the side of the *Herald of Free Enterprise* above the portholes which have been smashed to provide access to those trapped inside.

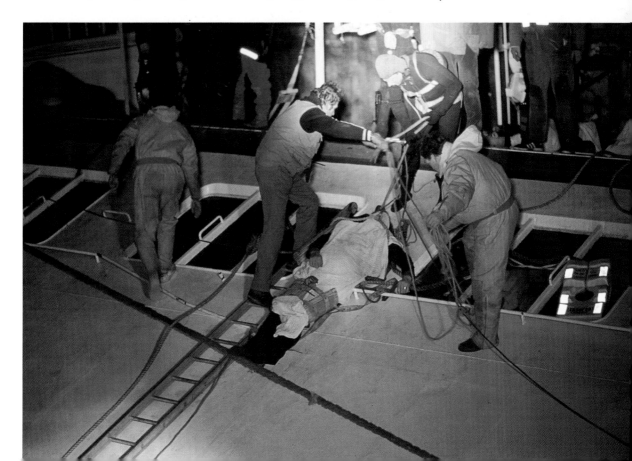

their clasped hands, and in this way, he got out. He found a small boy standing on the side of the ship alone and scooped him up into his arms, then the boy's father emerged with his pregnant wife whom he had gone back to rescue, having told the boy to stay exactly where he was. Stephen Homewood then started to organise rescue work, breaking windows, then helping people through them. When he saw people in the interior who could not climb out, he went back inside to help a Belgian Navy diver who was keeping survivors afloat in an area where many of them could not climb up the rope ladders. Homewood made several trips up and down again, pulling and pushing and exhorting people to get up and out to safety. Ropes were lowered into the darkness and he and the diver tied them round people who were then pulled to safety. One of them was Stan Mason, still with his baby Kerry gripped by her clothes in his teeth. A rope was lowered and Kerry tied to it, then pulled up from above. They pulled too hard and she was banged against the side of the ship. But she survived, as did her father.

Able Seaman Fullen from HMS *Hurworth* entered the ship with full diving gear strapped on. Inside the ferry, he found it far too restrictive, so he took off his mask and air bottles and sent them back to the surface on a rope, then swam through the ship. He stopped in various places, then he heard a sound, shouted for silence and found three lorry drivers alive in an air pocket.

When the ship rolled over, the Parker family – Andrew, a six-foot-two-inch ex-policeman, his wife Eleanor and their twelve-year-old daughter, Janice – were having a meal in the cafeteria. They were thrown across the room, but managed to stay together, landing in a huddle. The only route to safety was across a gap filled with water with barriers on either side. Andrew Parker braced himself against the barriers, forming a human bridge over the gap, and first his wife then Janice climbed over him, followed by around twenty other people who went out through a porthole. When the whole group was across, they hauled Andrew Parker up. Eleanor Parker was no longer there, she had already been taken off the ship.

There were less attractive stories. One female crew member, Jenny Leslie, managed to get her own life jacket on and handed out others to passengers. When there were none left, she took hers off and gave it to somebody who then brushed past her, pushing her into the water.

In another part of the ship, on another rope ladder, a man was clinging to it unable to move up or down through either shock or hypothermia or both. Underneath, in the freezing water were others who could use the ladder to save themselves. An Army Corporal, Peter Williamson, took a bold decision, shouting to those nearest to knock the man off the ladder. Others shouted the same instruction and those at the bottom shook it until he fell off into the water.

HMS *Hurworth* put to sea within forty-five minutes of the Mayday being received and arrived close by. Sub Lieutenant John Cox went on to the hull of the *Herald* where he organised a methodical plan to search through all the parts of the ship which could possibly be reached. Most of the survivors got out through the windows on the starboard side, many of them pulled up on ropes by those on top. It was exhausting work. Gradually the rescue services took over, as the crew and survivors who had helped became too exhausted and went by tug to the shore.

The death toll mounted, but the stream of survivors was steadily increasing too through the night thanks to the efforts of those working on the side of the ship. Many of the ship's crew had died; some simply survived by chance, but many instinctively put the lives of passengers first and undoubtedly among them some died in the process.

Blues and Twos

Opposite: The *Herald of Free Enterprise* as salvage begins. Eighty-one people were still not accounted for when the rescue was called off.

Below: There was universal praise for the speedy response of the Belgian authorities to the emergency: thirty ambulances were on hand to take survivors to hospital, hundreds of blankets were provided and few survivors spent longer than a minute on the quayside before being taken to hospital.

On the quayside, teams of doctors and nurses prioritised the survivors, many arriving in wet clothes and wrapped in blankets. Many had broken bones from being thrown about violently as the ship went over. Most were suffering from the extreme cold and from shock. Eventually there were over 100 ambulances delivering people to hospitals along the coast. Those without injury went to hotels and to Belgian Army quarters. The injured were taken to hospital in Zeebrugge and Bruges. The dead were taken to a temporary mortuary. As is so often the case in major disasters, sightseers flocked to the coast in cars to watch the rescue from the shore and created traffic jams in the process.

The last survivors were taken off in the early hours of Saturday morning. By daylight, there was little hope of finding any more people alive, though the grim task of bringing out the bodies went on. RAF Sea Kings continued to scan the wreck using thermal imaging cameras to detect any signs of life, but there were none, and search turned to recovering the dead.

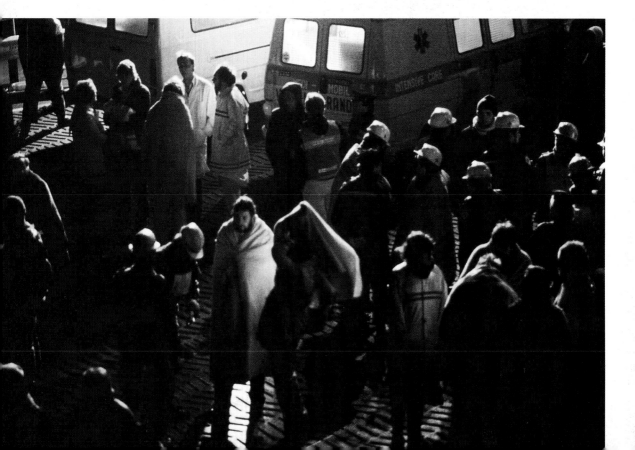

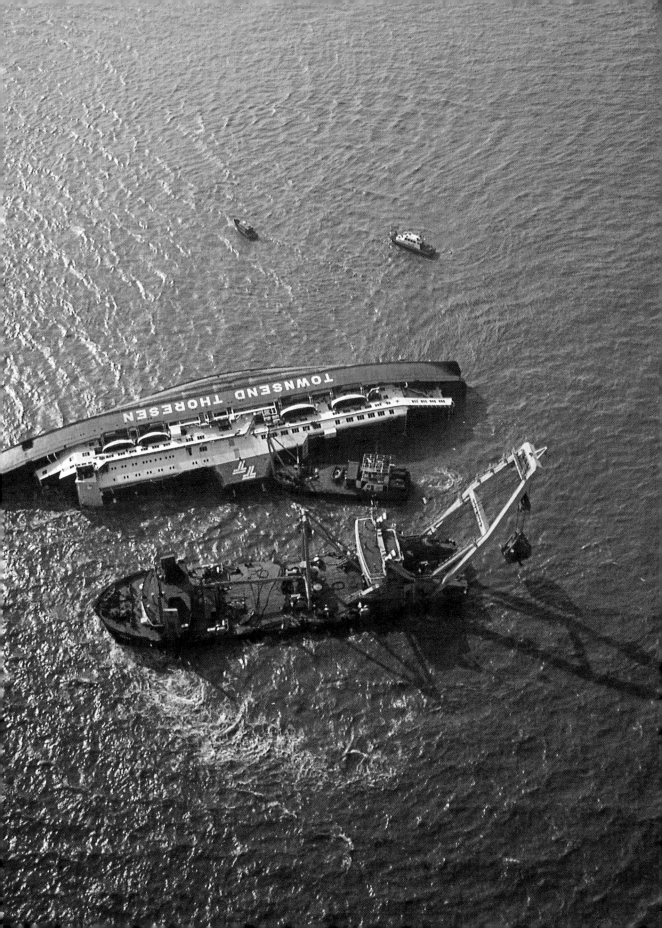

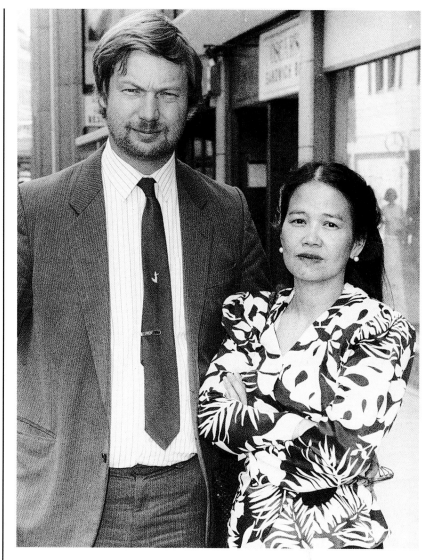

Hero of the *Herald of Free Enterprise* capsizing was Andrew Parker, aged thirty-three, seen here with his wife Eleanor. A former policeman, he formed a human bridge over a stairway so that others could escape.

It was a long time before some families were reunited with loved ones. Eleanor and Janice Parker were reunited in hospital in Belgium but they had to wait some time before they were told that Andrew had survived too. A special flight was arranged for the survivors, Flight BR 995 to Gatwick on Sunday 8 March with 190 survivors, including Martin Hartley.

There were 408 survivors and 193 died, thirty-eight of them

crew members. It was Britain's worst maritime disaster in peace time since the *Titanic* sank in 1912. The deaths were due to drowning but many were caused by hypothermia too. It was one of the biggest rescues mounted in peace time and it was mounted quickly and with great effect.

The popularity of going on foreign holidays has grown since the Second World War, not only by sea but in the air. Until the 1960s, flying had always been the preserve of the very rich, politicians and government servants. In the 1950s, the first holiday flights were pioneered in Britain by charter airlines who bought aircraft which the major airlines re-equipped with jets. Flights were organised by clubs or groups of people who could fill the whole aircraft, keeping the price of each seat low. On 12 March 1950, an Avro Tudor, owned by Fairflight and which had been used in the Berlin airlift, crashed while approaching Cardiff airport on its way back from Dublin. It was full of Welsh supporters who had been to the Wales versus Ireland rugby international. Three people survived, but eighty were killed, the worst toll in civil aviation's history.

Statistically, flying is a very safe way to travel, but when accidents happen they tend to involve a high percentage of fatalities because of the speed at which they occur, the fragility of the aircraft, and the way the passengers are tightly packed and in close proximity to the fuel and engines. Airports have their own specially trained fire and ambulance services, but saving people from air crashes is at the very limits of rescue techniques. On 8 April 1968, a BOAC Boeing 707 took off from London's Heathrow airport, but within minutes of becoming airborne, one of the engines on the port side caught fire and fell off. The captain made an emergency landing and as the aircraft came to a halt, a stewardess, Barbara Harrison, and a steward inflated the escape chute from the rear door, but it twisted as it opened and the steward had to go down to

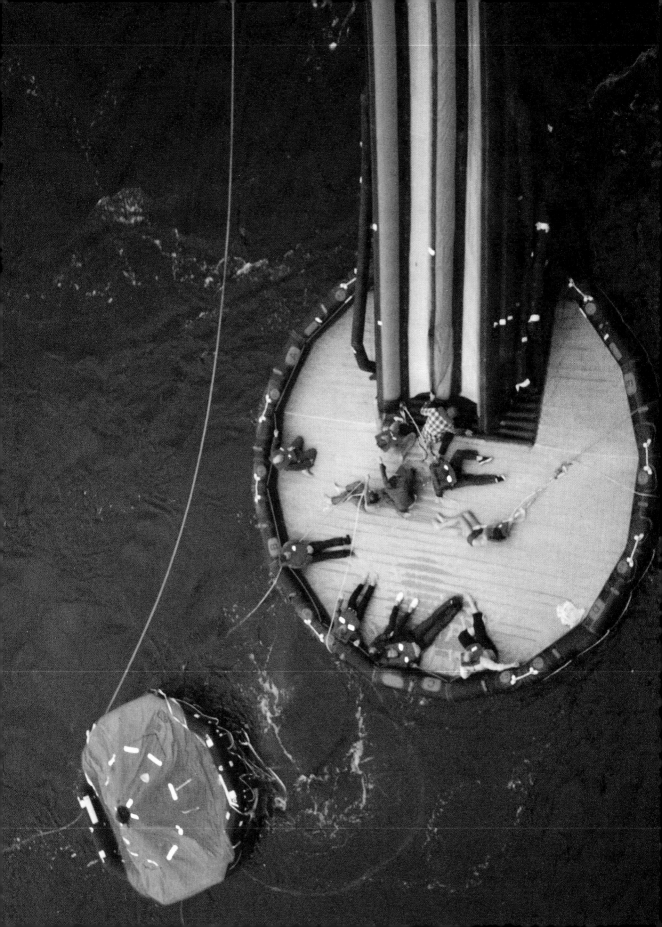

make it safe. Fire fighters were on the scene soon after the aircraft came to rest, but the fire spread rapidly in the fully fuelled aircraft. Barbara Harrison started organising the passengers to evacuate down the chute, urging some and pushing those who were reluctant, but as the fire intensified, the rear chute became unusable so she directed the remainder in her charge to another exit. She then began to help a disabled passenger who was still seated in one of the rear seats, but both of them were overcome by fumes and died in the aircraft. Barbara Harrison was posthumously awarded the George Cross.

The volume of flights and the size of aircraft have grown enormously in the 1960s, much of the increase the result of package holidays in the sun. Barely a year has gone by without some accident. On 18 June 1972, a BEA Trident had just taken off from Heathrow for Brussels when it suddenly crashed without warning in a field near Staines. Rescuers were on the scene quickly and put out a small fire which had started. They even brought one man out alive though he died later. All 118 people on the aircraft died, including the captain who had had a heart attack shortly after take-off.

The worst accident in aviation history was on 27 March 1977. Just as a KLM Boeing 747 was taking off from Las Palmas airport in the Canary Islands, a Pan American 747 turned on to the runway right across its path. The two aircraft collided; both were fully fuelled and they burst into flames. Fire tenders and ambulances rushed to the scene and there was an immediate appeal for doctors and nurses to go to their hospitals to receive the wounded, but 574 people died and the seventy survivors were very badly burned.

On 9 January 1989, a brand new British Midland Boeing 737 took off from Heathrow for Belfast with 117 passengers and eight crew on board. Shortly after take-off a fire started in the port engine, but the captain mistakenly closed down the starboard

Opposite: On 28 September 1994 the roll on–roll off ferry *Estonia* was en route from Tallinn to Stockholm when severe weather in the Gulf of Finland broke open the front loading doors. The *Estonia* sank very quickly and over 800 people lost their lives. The survivors in this photograph are being picked up by passenger ferry *Silja Symphony.*

Manchester Airport 22 August 1986: a Boeing 737 fully laden for a holiday flight to Corfu lost a turbine blade from its port engine on take off; it punctured fuel tanks and caught fire. The pilot managed to abort the take off, but fifty-four people died before the rescue services could enter the aircraft; seventy-nine were saved.

engine. He prepared to make an emergency landing at the East Midlands airport near Nottingham, but as he approached, he had too little power and crashed just short of the runway on the embankment of the M1 motorway.

Police closed off the motorway as the fire and ambulance services rushed to the scene. The fuselage of the 737 was broken in several places giving the rescuers a way in to the tangled mixture of people and wreckage. First on the scene was Maurice Foster, a paramedic with the Derbyshire Ambulance Service, and his colleague Jim Gough. They immediately radioed that the crash was a major incident, putting all local hospitals on alert, then set about treating the survivors. Once again, the speed of getting skilled medical staff to the site saved lives. It was five hours before all the survivors were taken out. Had there been a fire, the task would

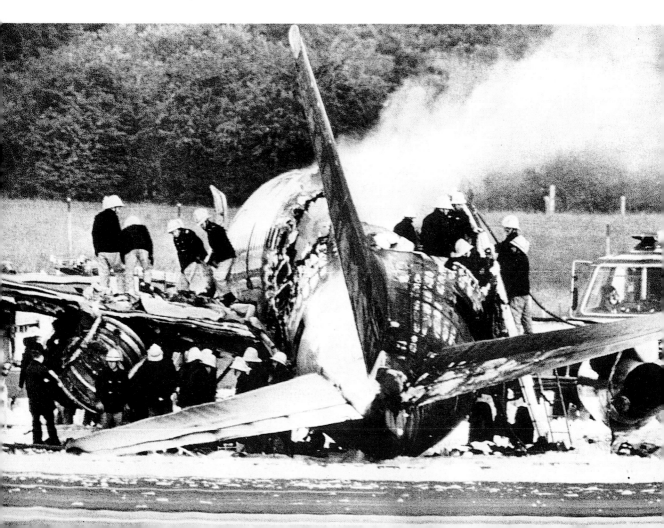

have been much more difficult, but of the 125 people on board, seventy-eight survived, including the captain – an extraordinary tribute to the rescuers.

Travel by land, sea and air continues to increase, and the personal tragedies which accompany the train crashes, ferry disasters and air crashes still happen. But though they make the headlines, major transport disasters are by definition the exception rather than the rule. By far and away the most frequent type of incident that the emergency services attend arises from what has become the symbol of personal mobility – and also the biggest killer – the motor car, which is now at the heart of the transport system. Britain's first motorway, the M1, was opened on 2 November 1959, and the network of motorways which followed opened up unprecedented opportunities to travel and with them an inexorable rise in the numbers of cars on Britain's roads. Unfortunately that has resulted in a steady rise in the number of deaths and injuries on the roads.

The rise in fatalities peaked in the late 1960s and 1970s, prompting legislation to clamp down on drinking and driving and to enforce the compulsory wearing of seat belts. There have been some huge multiple crashes on Britain's motorways, the first just a month after the M1 was opened, caused mainly by people driving too fast in either foggy or icy conditions. In many cases, the accidents were made far worse by cars and trucks ploughing into the stationary vehicles, sometimes even after the emergency services had arrived. Police patrol the motorways, and all three emergency services have routine plans to cope with major road traffic accidents. Over the years of dealing with crashes the need for visibility has become paramount. Flashing blue lights and full-length fluorescent jackets both owe their existence to the men and women of the fire, police and ambulance services wanting to be seen on motorways. Britain is one of the safest countries in the world to

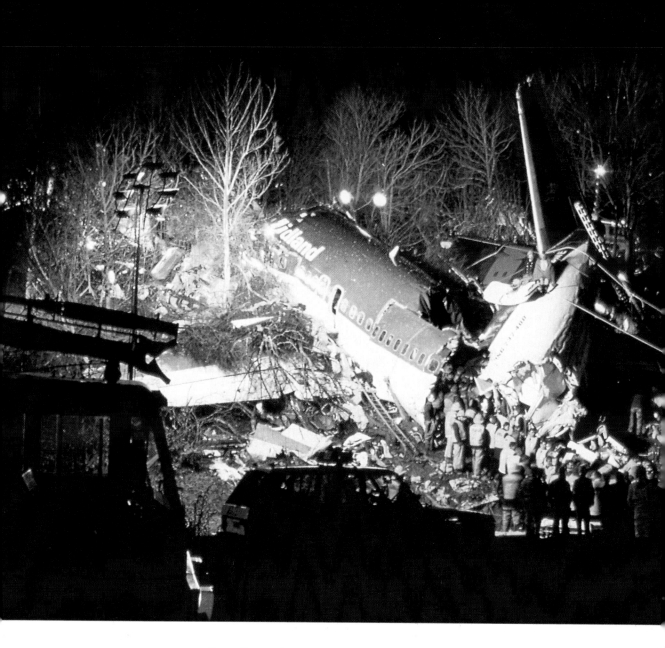

drive in, and its motorways are among the safest roads, but even so, around 5000 people are killed and over 300,000 people are injured on Britain's roads every year. In most of those accidents the toll would have been higher but for the prompt action and skills of the emergency services. But even after years of experience in dealing with them, they remain one of the most harrowing and stressful experiences for police, fire and ambulance officers. Treating small children with bandages and saline drips as they are cut out of crumbled and burned family cars takes toughness, both physical and psychological. If the child lives it is one of the best jobs in the world; if they die it is the worst, especially when someone has to tell relatives – often part of the daily routine of doctors and nurses in casualty departments.

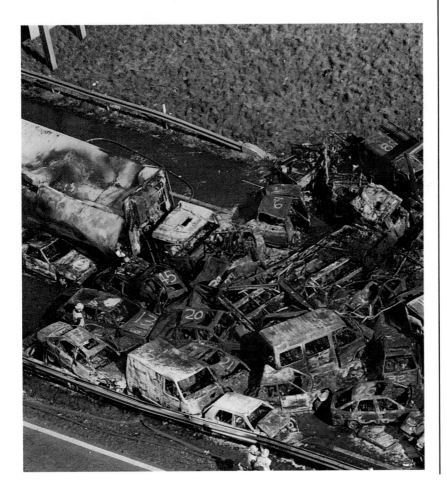

Opposite: The emergency services arrived quickly when a British Midland Boeing 737 crashed into the embankment of the M1 motorway just short of the runway at East Midlands Airport near Nottingham on 9 January 1989; they saved seventy-nine of the 125 people on board.

Left: Motorway pile-ups, such as this one on the M-4, make the news because they often involve large numbers of casualties. In truth motorways are among our safest roads and despite increases in the number of, and use of, cars over the last twenty years, motorways have contributed to an overall decline in the number of Road Traffic Accidents (RTAs). Since 1970, deaths in RTAs have been reduced from 7,500 to 4,200, a fall of 44 per cent, and the total number of casualties has fallen from 363,000 to 310,000.

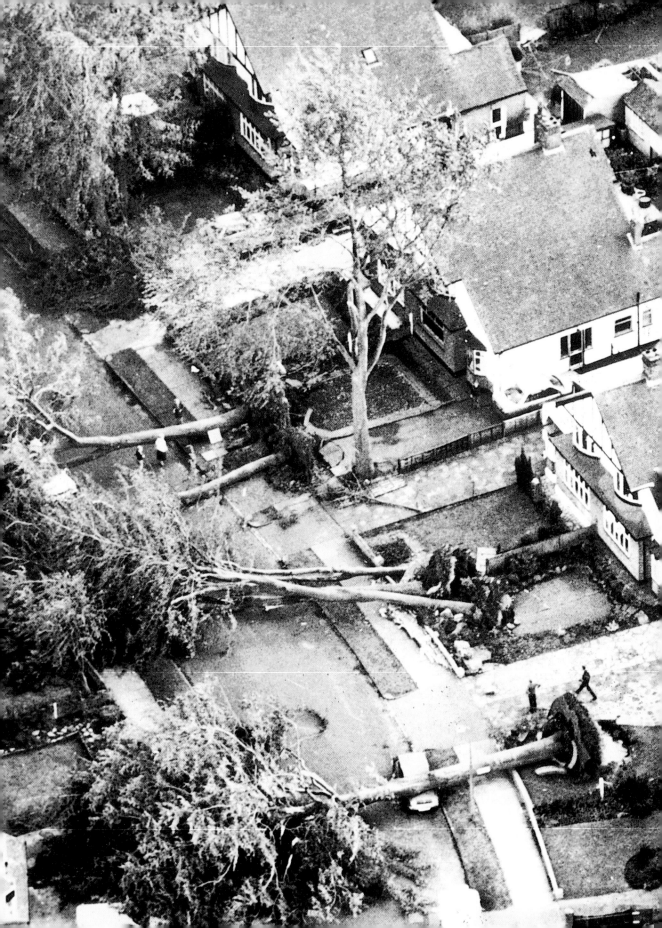

Chapter Seven

STORM FORCE

On 12 October 1987, the European Centre for Medium Range Weather Forecasting at Reading in Berkshire, one of the most advanced in the world, issued a warning of very high winds from the Atlantic in four days' time. While Britain was enjoying quite mild weather, out in the middle of the moody ocean it was very cold, and the difference between the two areas would result in a very severe depression which would move across southern England and northern France. The French Meteorological Office checked the data and acted on it, issuing severe weather warnings to the people in the north of the country through radio and television broadcasts. The French broadcasts were picked up by some people in southern England who telephoned the London Weather Centre to make enquiries, but even at 9 o'clock on Thursday evening, 15 October, the centre's tape-recorded message was still forecasting 'a cool, dry day' though 'winds will be quite strong'.

The Meteorological Office's computers suggested that it would not be a severe storm and what there was of it, the computers predicted, would pass broadly up the English Channel out of harm's way. That night, the BBC weatherman Ian McCaskill was equally relaxed, giving no indication of anything serious in the offing. The

Opposite: The morning after the Great Storm of October 1987, residents of Orpington in Kent woke up to find many of the trees which lined their leafy estate flattened and their cars crushed by hurricane force winds.

189

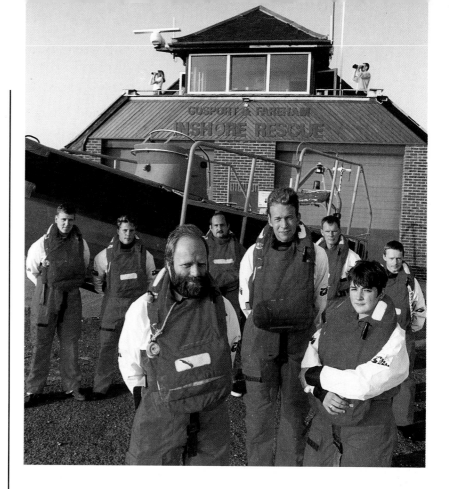

Volunteers: the crew of the Gosport and Fareham Inshore Rescue Service (GAFIRS) featured in the first series of *Blues and Twos* on one of their busiest days, in June 1994, during the celebrations to mark the fiftieth anniversary of D-Day. From left to right: Stuart Pattison, Mike Davies, Colin Pipe, Ken Pink (coxswain), John Donne, Jane King, Mike Allen and Andy Hillier; with binoculars, Emma Adolpho and Paul Waugh.

country went to bed as usual: no alerts were sent to local authorities or to the emergency services who made no special arrangements.

Shortly after 9 o'clock, atmospheric pressure began to drop suddenly and deeply as the storm veered towards central England and by midnight it had sunk to a record low of 957 millibars. The first warning to the country that the situation had changed came at 12.20a.m. after the late news on BBC Radio Four, by which time winds were already reaching Force 11, violent storm, just one point below hurricane force on the Beaufort Scale.

The path of the storm was straight across southern England, from Cornwall to East Anglia. It wreaked havoc along a swathe of the country 100 miles wide. Gusts of 110mph blew over trees which landed on cars and people; tore down scaffolding; blew down chimneys; stripped the cladding off the exteriors of high-rise buildings and the tiles and slates off many roofs; and brought down electricity pylons like matchsticks – three million people were eventually without electricity.

Members of the emergency services responded as quickly as they could. Between 1 and 3a.m., the London Ambulance Service answered 155 999 calls, mainly taking to hospital people who had been injured by falling trees and those relying on respirators whose equipment had been cut off by power cuts. In the next twenty-four hours, the London Fire Service answered 6000 999 rescue calls, twice the previous record and against a daily average of 350. The problems that they faced were mainly to free people with minor injuries who had been trapped in damaged houses. Police supervised the evacuation of high-rise blocks of flats as they suffered structural damage.

In Hampshire, a part-time fire crew which had just finished

The Sealink ferry *Hengist*, blown ashore at Folkstone after putting to sea in the Great Storm to make room for another ferry, with passengers on board, to enter the harbour. All the crew members of the *Hengist* were rescued.

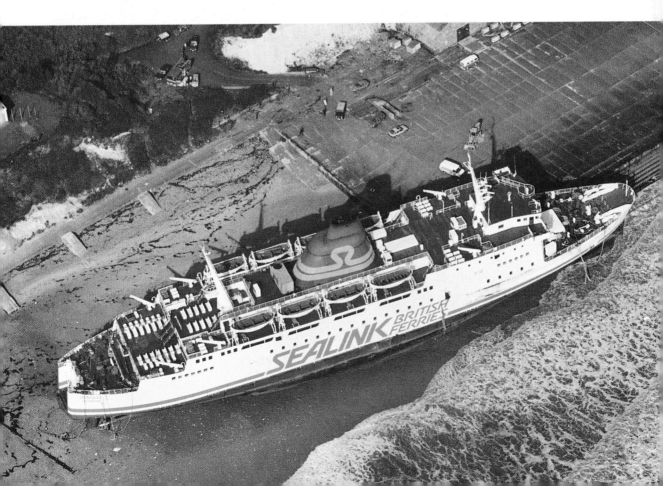

securing the roof to a church in Christchurch then answered a call to a factory where the fire alarm had gone off. As they drove through Highcliffe, a tree crashed down on to the cab, killing Sub Officer Ernest Gregory and Fireman Graham White. The call turned out to be a false alarm, one of thousands of fire and burglar alarms set off by the storm.

In the North Sea, off Cromer in Norfolk, helicopters had to lift the men off several gas rigs, flying in 80mph winds. In the Channel, the bulk carrier *Sumneo* overturned just outside Dover harbour, blocking the entrance. The Dover lifeboat was launched and managed to save four of the crew and a Sea King helicopter from RAF Manston searched the area for two more, but they were drowned.

The Weymouth lifeboat was called out to rescue the crew of a catamaran off Portland, and the Royal Navy destroyer HMS *Birmingham* went to help .The waves around the stricken craft were too high for the lifeboat to approach, so the destroyer's crew poured diesel fuel on to the water to calm it down – literally oil on troubled waters – as the lifeboat went in to rescue the crew of six.

The seas off the south-east coast were too high for car ferries to approach their harbours, so 900 passengers were stranded on two ships, one trying to get into Harwich, the other into Dover; they had to ride out the storm in huge seas for twelve hours.

The captain of the Sealink car ferry *St Christopher* with 150 passengers had no warning of the storm as he left Calais at 3a.m. for a ninety-minute journey to Dover, but the overturned *Sumneo* was blocking the harbour entrance so they had to stay at sea in forty-foot waves, water crashing into the car deck, turning over trucks and cars. The ship finally arrived in Dover at 2 o'clock on Friday afternoon. The crew of the Sealink ferry *Hengist* took her to sea to make way in the harbour for another ferry which had to dock with passengers. The winds, gusting over 100mph, were too much for the ferry and it was blown up on a beach near Folkestone where the twenty-two men were rescued by breeches-buoy. In a sad postscript, the hulk of the Townsend Thorensen ferry *Herald of Free Enterprise*, which had overturned at Zeebrugge, was being towed to a breaker's yard in Taiwan and snapped its tow line in the Bay of Biscay and drifted in the storm.

Rail services were brought to a virtual standstill by hundreds of trees across the lines. The Stock Exchange ceased functioning because there were too few people available to man the switchboards. When a block of flats started to collapse in Brighton the residents had to be evacuated. The Isle of Wight's famous Shanklin pier fell into the sea with all its amusement booths. The collection of trees at Kew Gardens was flattened. In the Channel Islands acres and acres of glass houses were destroyed. The final cost was put at over £300 million.

Eighteen people in the United Kingdom lost their lives in the Great Storm, most of them killed by falling trees or masonry; in France four people died. It was the worst storm recorded since 1703, when a reported 8000 people died. It was a prime example of how modern society can place too much faith in sophisticated technology and become complacent about the forces of nature, which are truly awesome. But once again it showed how that society with its emergency services was able to respond. It is impossible to say how many people were saved, but without the network of 999 telephones linking police, fire, ambulance, RAF and RN rescue helicopters and the RNLI, the death toll would have been much higher.

Of all the pieces of technology which have been used for humanitarian purposes, especially when it comes to rescuing people from the forces of nature, probably the most significant is the helicopter. The first practical helicopter was built during the Second World War in America by Igor Sikorski, a Russian emigré living in New

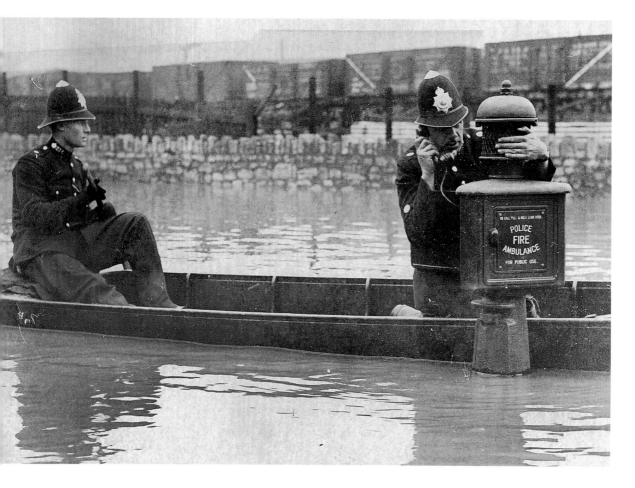

In March 1947, Britain was hit by severe storms which resulted in flooding in many parts of the country; in Bath, Somerset, police used boats to deliver food to elderly people, keeping in touch with base using the emergency telephone system.

York. The first time it was used was to save life in Burma: three wounded British soldiers were being airlifted by a USAAF single-engined light aircraft out of the Burmese jungle. The engine failed and the pilot, Sergeant Ernst Hladovkak, made a forced landing behind Japanese lines. A tiny experimental air unit was attached to the US Air Forces supporting the soldiers and equipped with three R-4 Sikorski helicopters. The four men had come down beyond the range of the R-4, but they stayed in the jungle for five days while plans were made to evacuate them. Lieutenant Carter Harman managed to adapt his R-4 by strapping an extra fuel tank on the top of the cockpit giving him the range to reach them. The payload of the R-4 was one pilot, but Harman managed to lift them out one at a time to an improvised airstrip in a dried-up river bed not far away, where an L-5 fixed-wing aircraft could land and fly them to hospital.

In the same year, on 29 November 1945, violent storms drove an oil barge on to rocks just off the coast in Long Island Sound with two crew on board. A Sikorski R-5 flown by Dmitri Viner, a nephew of the designer, flew out in 60mph winds. Sikorski had always emphasised the humanitarian potential of the helicopter and he had equipped the R-5 with a winch operated by a second crew man. They winched the first man off, but had to fly him to the shore since the helicopter could only carry three people, then go back for the other. When he was halfway up, the winch jammed and he had to be flown ashore dangling underneath, the first time a hoist was used to lift survivors. The age of the rescue helicopter was born, but it took many years before they had the range and lifting capacity which they have today.

The primary function of RAF and Royal Navy rescue helicopters is to rescue aircrew from downed aircraft in both peace and war, but over the years, the cover they have offered for civilian rescue has been incorporated into the national emergency service. This cover is not only at sea but in mountain areas, where specialist techniques, flying close to rock faces to rescue climbers, where the wind comes off the mountains in unpredictable gusts, have been developed to a very high level. The RN and RAF rescue services are highly valued by the public, and whenever cost cutting has hit the Ministry of Defence, and there are possibilities of cutbacks, public pressure keeps them in civilian service. It is a very secure feeling to know that there are airmen, with the same values and courage as the RNLI, ready to go out in any weather when there are people in distress.

One such occasion came in August 1979. Every other year since 1925, except for the war years, a yacht race has been run from

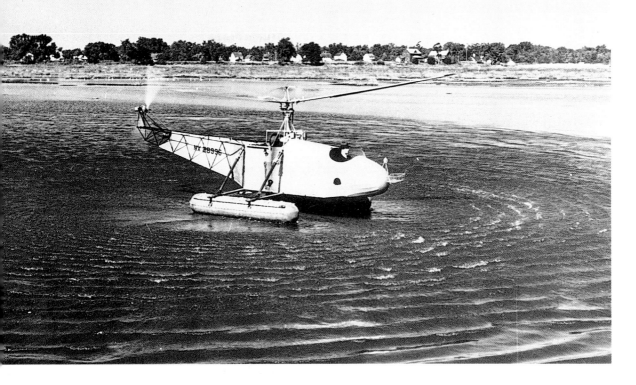

Birth of the perfect rescue machine: an early Sikorski helicopter demonstrating its versatility on water in 1945. Developed for war, the helicopter swiftly established itself as a valuable aid to humanitarian work.

Cowes, as part of Cowes Week, round Land's End to the Fastnet Rock off southern Ireland and back – a distance of around 600 miles. It takes the fastest yachts about three to four days and the slowest about a week. On the afternoon of Saturday 11 August, 303 yachts set out in fine weather, but by late on the night of Monday 13 August, the weather was deteriorating by the hour as a huge storm brewed up, reaching Hurricane Force 11 at its height. By late evening there were numerous reports coming in from yachts taking part in the race that they were in trouble, many of them losing rudders. They were stretched out across 150 miles of sea between Land's End and Ireland, and after midnight there were numerous reports of red flares being sent up and Mayday calls being made. At 10.15p.m., the Baltimore lifeboat in south-west Ireland was launched to tow in the first victim, then between midnight and 3 o'clock in the morning four more lifeboats were launched from Ireland and together with a fishery patrol vessel, HMS *Anglesey*, they were sent to the area to assist the race guard ship, the Dutch destroyer HNMLS *Overijssel*.

Because it was still dark, air searches were delayed until dawn, but an RAF Nimrod maritime patrol aircraft took off from Scotland and arrived over the race area at 5.30a.m. to act as an airborne command post for the mounting rescue effort. The first helicopter, a Navy Wessex, call sign Rescue 20, took off from Culdrose at 4.35a.m., followed almost immediately by a Sea King, Rescue 77. By now there were four yachts in serious difficulty: *Mulligatawny*, *Magic*, *Grimalkin* and *Tarantula* which had reported that it was sinking at 5.18a.m.

Rescue 77 arrived overhead the *Tarantula* at 7.45a.m. to find the mast was whipping back and forth so fiercely that the winch could not be used. Over a VHF radio link the pilot told the crew to jump

Royal Navy Wessex helicopter, Rescue 27, rescuing a crew member of the yacht *Carmargue* which they had to abandon during the Fastnet Race in 1979.

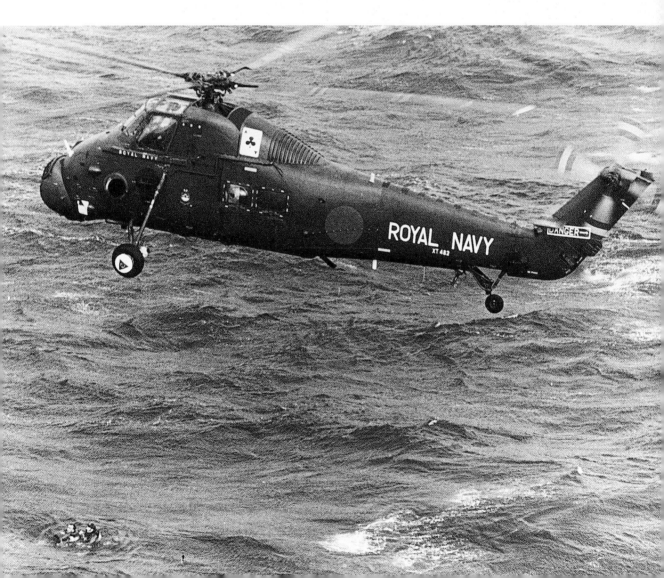

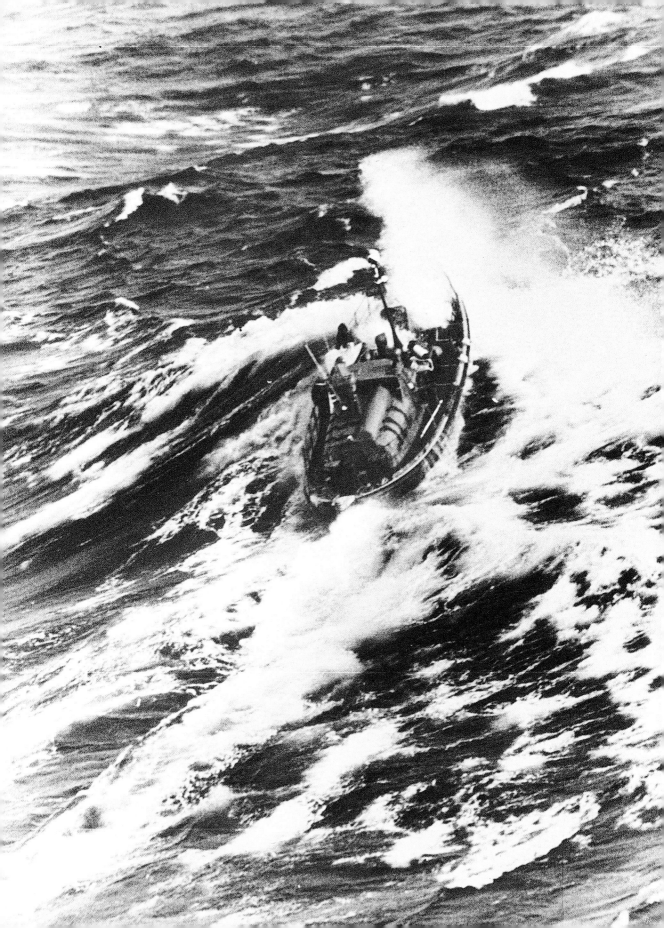

into the sea, one by one, and swim away from the yacht where they would be picked up. The first to jump was Jacques Souben but it took half an hour to winch him up and the rest of the crew decided to wait for a surface vessel and they were eventually picked up by a French trawler.

Rescue 20 found *Magic* after a long and difficult search in forty-foot waves. Again, it was impossible to use the winch because of the swinging mast, so the five crew jumped into the sea and were lifted up one by one by the winchman, Leading Aircraftman Grinney, and flown back to Culdrose. Rescue 97 picked up two survivors from the *Trophy*.

For many of the yachtsmen it was difficult to decide whether to stay with a stricken vessel or abandon it for life rafts. In the *Grimalkin* the crew of six were being thrown about fiercely in the cockpit, and on one occasion the yacht was thrown right over until the mast touched the sea and they were thrown out. They clambered back in but two of them were severely injured. Then the boat overturned completely and the skipper, David Sheahan, was trapped underneath. The other crew members cut him free, then the boat was righted by the weather, but Sheahan was swept away and drowned. With two others unconscious, the three survivors decided to abandon her, and took to an inflatable dinghy. They were rescued by another Sea King.

Royal Navy and RAF helicopters with spare crews from other parts of Britain arrived at Culdrose to assist the search, and two Nimrods circled overhead coordinating their efforts. Sometimes the Nimrods flew low and spotted the wrecks, then guided the helicopters to them to make the rescue. So it went on throughout the day and into the next: yachtsmen were washed overboard, some scrambling back on board their dismasted, wallowing boats using their lifelines, others being washed away; some jumping into the sea and being rescued by helicopters, only to die from hypothermia on

Opposite: The Scilly Isles lifeboat at sea during the Fastnet Race searching for victims of the storms.

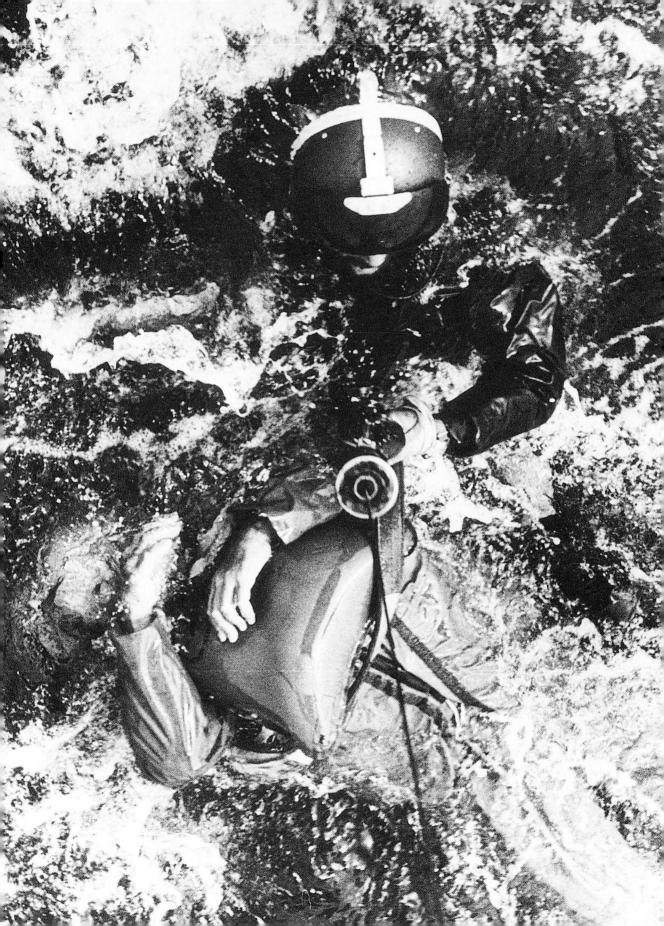

the way to hospital; five men from the *Ariadne* took to their dinghy, but three of them were lost when they fell into the sea while trying to transfer to a German ship.

The death toll for the first day was fifteen, but seventy-five people were rescued by helicopter, the last at 7.25 in the evening, and another sixty-five by surface vessels. Thirteen lifeboats were launched in the course of the following three days and the search for survivors went on until every yacht which had weathered the storm was accounted for. Only eighty-five yachts completed the race which was won by the American TV tycoon, Ted Turner.

On 11 August 1985 the weather off Cornwall was appalling, Force 9 winds and driving rain. In the early morning a Mayday call was received by the Coastguard from a yacht, the *Mister Cube*, which was stranded fifty-five miles off the Lizard with its jib blown away and an auxiliary engine which would not start. On board were three adults and six children. At the Royal Naval Air Station at Culdrose, a Search and Rescue Wessex took off into weather which was only just within the flying limits, a low cloud base and fierce rain squalls. The pilot was Lieutenant David Marr, the winch operator Petty Officer Michael Palmer, and the diver–winchman was Petty Officer Larry Slater. They had no radar, so had to find the yacht by dead reckoning. When they did find her, she was being pounded by twenty-five-foot seas and rolling through 90 degrees, the masts whipping back and forth, while also rising and falling in the swell.

The rescue crew's first idea was a hi-line rescue, a technique which involves dropping a weighted line from the helicopter to the deck for somebody on board to grab. The line then acts as a guide through all the rigging and masts, helps the pilot to hover in the right place over the stricken vessel, and can be used to winch the survivors to the helicopter. Slater then went down on the winch

Opposite: Royal Navy winchman/diver Petty Officer Roy Henshaw preparing to lift the owner of the yacht *Ariadne*, Frank Ferris, from the Irish Sea during the Fastnet Race. Ferris died on the way to hospital.

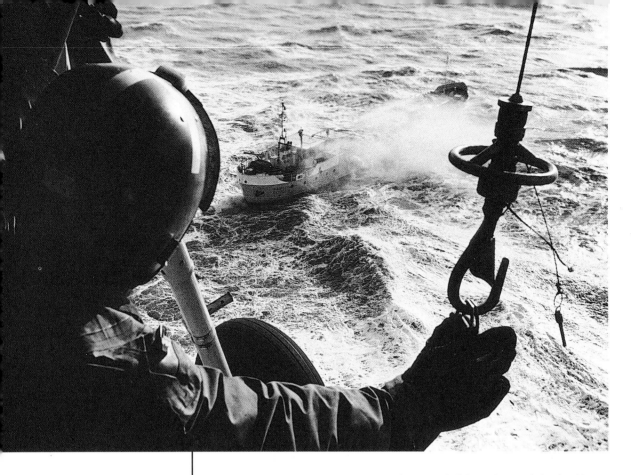

A Search and Rescue (SAR) helicopter from RAF Manston approaching the German coaster *Warfleth* which ran aground on a sandbank off the Kent coast during a storm in January 1979. RAF and Royal Navy helicopters have been based around the coast of Britain since they first came into service in the 1950s, combining their military duties with an SAR service to civilians.

to supervise the adults and the larger children being lifted off one by one, then he would go up with the smaller children. The first two of the adults then went up on their own when a wave hit the *Mister Cube* putting her on her side. The helicopter had to be repositioned, then the lift started again and the remaining crew were lifted off and flown to Culdrose.

At 2p.m. the same day, another call came through from the Coastguard reporting a capsized yacht, the *Drum England*, one of the contestants in that year's Fastnet race, which had overturned a mile and a half offshore at Porthscatho. When they arrived overhead, the helicopter crew saw eighteen people sitting on the upturned hull indicating that there were still people trapped inside. Larry Slater jumped from the helicopter into the sea, then swam to the side of the yacht to speak to those on top who told him that six men were still trapped inside. Slater carried breathing apparatus and quickly dived under the yacht, picking his way through the rigging, booms and sails until he found a hatch. He was not sure it was in the right place, so returned to check with the people on the hull who confirmed it was. Back he went, opened the hatch and found six men inside, including Simon Le Bon, the singer in the Duran Duran pop group and owner of the *Drum England*. They were standing up to their waists in water mixed with fuel and battery acid and the air pocket was laced with fuel vapour and fumes. Slater decided to go back to the helicopter for breathing apparatus for them, but when he returned yet again, he decided that it was too bulky for them to operate while swimming, so instead he told them to take deep breaths and took each one out and on to the hull. From the hull, twenty survivors were winched to the Wessex, while four were taken of by the Falmouth lifeboat.

The two rescues on the same day, especially one of them of a pop idol, received wide publicity. Petty Officer Slater was awarded the George Medal for his part in the two rescues. As an individual act of bravery his actions stood out, but the *Mister Cube* rescue was infinitely more difficult for the whole crew technically, and Lieutenant Marr and Petty Officer Palmer were both awarded the Queen's Commendation for Valuable Service in the Air.

Rescues from storms at sea have a particularly humane quality: stories of being plucked from the certainty of a lonely, cold and slow death by a stranger prepared to share that danger are as moving as they are exciting. For nearly two centuries, lifeboat crews have never failed to challenge even the most dangerous seas for the lives of those in distress and there are many heroic stories in the annals of the RNLI. Here are just two which embrace a living tradition which must never be taken for granted.

On 2 December 1966, the Coastguard informed the Holyhead lifeboat that a Greek ship, the *Nafsiporos*, had broken down twenty miles off the north-west coast of Anglesey and was wallowing in heavy seas which would eventually bring it on to rocks on the north coast of the island. The Douglas lifeboat had already been launched and was searching the area between Anglesey and the Isle of Man. Two RAF Shackleton maritime reconnaissance aircraft had also been called on to search the same area. The Holyhead lifeboat crew was summoned, and as they gathered at the boat house, they were joined by an RNLI Inspector, Lieutenant Commander Harold Harvey, who was in Anglesey making his annual inspection. It was agreed with the coxswain, Thomas Alcock, that he would come as extra crew on the *St Cybi*.

They set out in Storm Force 10 winds, and while they were sailing towards the search area, the Shackletons found the *Nafsiporos* fourteen miles from the Skerries, a rocky outcrop off the northeast coast of Anglesey. When the RAF pilots saw the *St Cybi*

A member of the *Warfleth* crew approaching the safety of an RAF Wessex SAR helicopter. The Wessex was the workhorse of Search and Rescue from the 1960s for over twenty years, but it has now been superseded by the larger, longer range and better equipped Sea King.

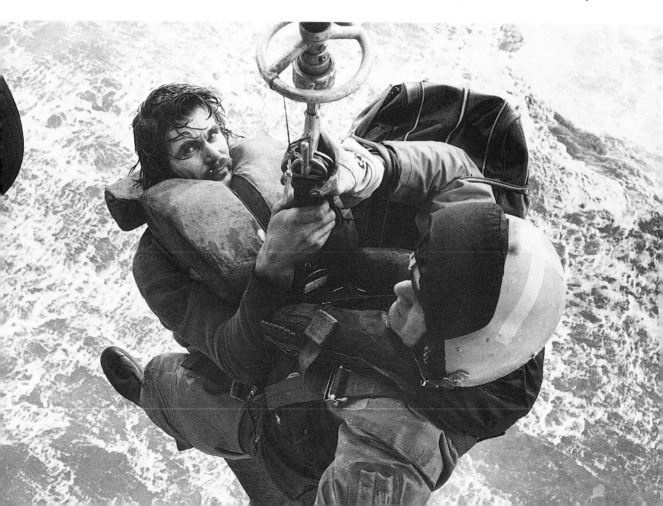

approaching, one of them flew towards it and guided it towards the stricken merchant ship.

The same morning, at Moelfre on the north coast of Anglesey, the lifeboat *Watkin Williams* had been launched to search the same general area for two other ships in distress: the *MV Vinland* and the *Grit*, whose steering gear had broken. The coxswain of the Moelfre boat was Richard Evans who had been awarded the RNLI Gold Medal in 1959 for rescuing eight men from the *Hindlea* before it broke up on rocks on the coast of Anglesey. He stood by to help the *Grit*, but the crew managed to jury rig a steering system and decided to weather the storm. Meanwhile a tug and another merchantman had found the *Vinland* and took her in tow, so Richard Evans returned to his base. Just as he got there, a call came through to join in the rescue of the *Nafsiporos*, so the crew put back to sea just after 2 o'clock into what were now hurricane force winds.

The engineless ship was now about eight miles from the shore and drifting towards Bull Bay at three and a half knots, rolling through 70 degrees. The two lifeboats stood by while a Russian vessel, the *Kungurles*, managed to get a tow line on board, but it parted soon afterwards. Then the captain of the *Nafsiporos* dropped anchor, but it failed to take hold and she was getting too close to the rocks with no room left for towing. The wind was gusting 120mph, visibility was very poor and just before 4 o'clock, the sun went down.

Coxswain Alcock of the *St Cybi* made the first attempt at getting alongside, coming round the stern just as the *Nafsiporos* rolled towards it and part of the superstructure hit the lifeboat and damaged it. The Greek crew then tried to launch one of their own lifeboats, but they let go the forward fall rope and it finished up hanging vertically by the stern rope, swinging wildly along the side of the ship. Unfortunately it was hanging just forward of the jumping ladder which would be used to evacuate the crew. The

The Greek merchant ship *Nafsiporos* adrift in hurricane force winds off the north coast of Anglesey in December 1966; three lifeboats, from the Isle of Man, Holyhead and Moelfre were launched and rescued most of the crew in one of the most remarkable rescues in the history of the RNLI.

lifeboatmen indicated to the crew that they should cut it free but they did not.

Richard Evans in the Moelfre lifeboat made the next attempt, but he too had to get out of the way in a hurry, in danger of being hit by the dangling lifeboat. Then he made another run and got alongside, but this time he was unable to persuade any of the crew to jump.

Meanwhile, Coxswain Alcock asked Lieutenant Commander Harvey to take the helm of the Holyhead boat so that he could take up a position in the bow which would normally have been filled by an experienced member of the crew who was ill that day and had not come on the rescue. What followed was one of the great achievements of the lifeboat service: Harvey edged in using the tide; there was a *Nafsiporos* crew member on the jumping ladder, but the swell was so high that at one moment he was out of reach below, then above. Harvey managed to get alongside at the right moment and the lifeboat crew pulled the man into the boat. Alcock

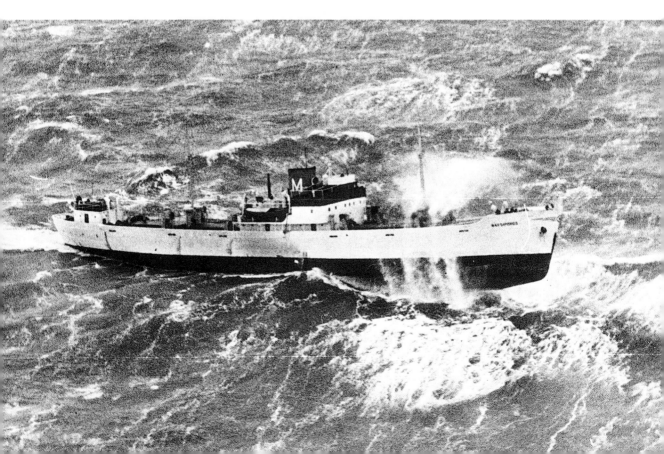

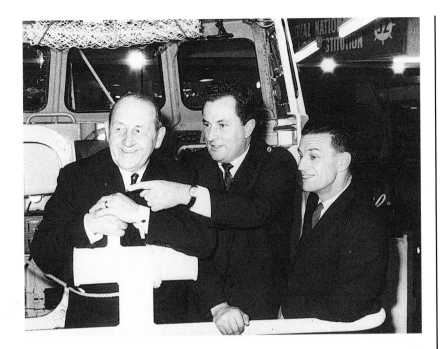

Heroes of the *Nafsiporos* rescue: Coxswain Richard Evans (left) and Lieutenant-Commander Harold Harvey (centre) were both awarded the RNLI Gold Medal for their parts in the *Nafsiporos* rescue, while Coxswain Thomas Alcock was awarded the society's Silver Medal.

was in charge of the rescue party while Harvey continued to handle the rising and falling lifeboat, enabling another four men to be grabbed, their confidence in the work of the lifeboat increasing each time. Once or twice, the *St Cybi* was hit by the swinging ship's lifeboat, and just as the fifth crew member was about to jump, the rear fall rope snapped and it came crashing down onto the deck of the Holyhead boat. In trying to avoid it, Harvey had used the engines to reverse away, and though it caused more damage, fortunately it slid off the port side.

The wreckage of the ship's lifeboat was now between the *Nafsiporos* and the Holyhead lifeboat, so Harvey pulled away and the Moelfre lifeboat took over once the wreckage had drifted away. Coxswain Evans and his crew managed to get another ten men off the same ladder, but the Greek captain and two men stayed on board.

The two RNLI lifeboats sailed back to Holyhead to drop off the fifteen men they had saved, but as soon as they had landed the

Opposite: The Penlee lifeboat *Solomon Browne* being launched in 1981; later in the year, the whole crew of eight was lost attempting to rescue the crew of the *Union Star.*

Holyhead boat went back to the *Nafsiporos* and stood by her through the night until a tug managed to get a line to her, the scene illuminated by flares dropped from RAF Shackletons flying overhead.

Even in the extraordinary annals of the RNLI it was an exceptional rescue, everything done with the traditional cool courage and disregard for their own lives by the crews. Lieutenant Commander Harvey and Coxswain Evans were both awarded the Gold Medal, Coxswain Alcock was awarded the Silver Medal with three other crew members, and a further twelve Bronze Medals were awarded to men of both crews.

On 19 December 1981, a brand new coaster, the *Union Star*, was on her maiden voyage with a cargo of fertiliser from Denmark, where she was built, to Dublin. There were eight people on board: the captain, Henry Moreton, his wife, and their two teenage daughters, plus four crew. Coming round Land's End around 6p.m., Moreton reported to the Coastguard that the *Union Star*'s main

Coxwain Trevelyan Richards, aged 56, of the Penlee lifeboat *Solomon Browne*, who died with his crew on 12 December 1981 off the coast of Cornwall going to the aid of the merchant ship *Union Star* in hurricane force winds. He was posthumously awarded the RNLI Gold Medal.

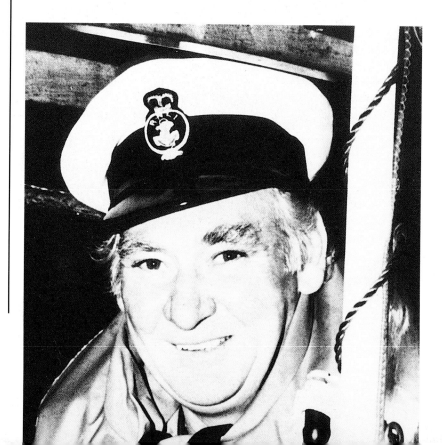

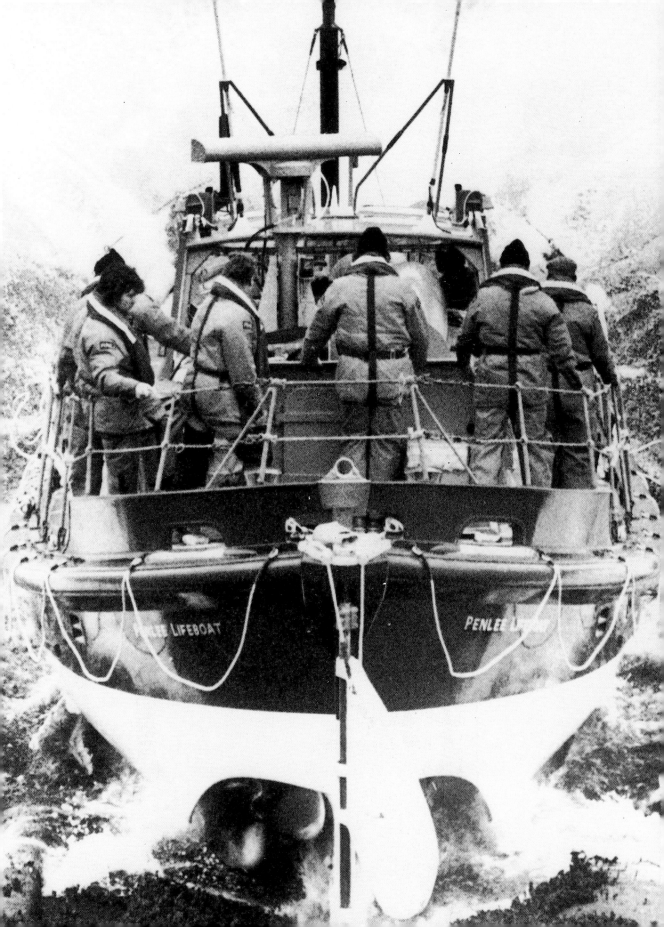

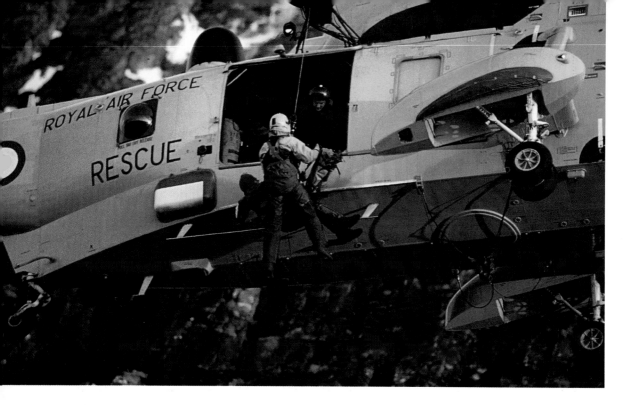

Mountain Rescue: an RAF Sea King rescue helicopter from Lossiemouth lifting a critically injured climber to safety after he and two colleagues were caught in an avalanche in the Cairngorms. Flying close to mountains calls for a very high level of skill to cope with sudden gusts of wind blowing off the mountains. Rescuing people from avalanches is especially tricky as the rotors can whip up fallen snow, covering the casualties.

engine had failed eight miles off Wolf Rock Lighthouse. Assistance under a Lloyd's contract was offered by Captain Johannes Buurman of the salvage tug *Noord Holland* which was in the port of Newlyn. Captain Moreton rejected the offer, but asked for a rescue helicopter to be put on standby and a Royal Navy Sea King was put on short notice at 6.15p.m. So was the Penlee lifeboat, the *Solomon Browne*, and its eight-man crew under Coxswain Trevelyan Richards, all of whom lived in the tiny fishing village of Mousehole. Captain Buurmans put to sea at 6.40p.m., into what he later described as the 'worst seas he had ever seen'.

In worsening weather, winds up to Force 12 and waves reaching sixty feet at their highest, the *Union Star* began drifting towards cliffs close to Land's End. Just after 7.30p.m., the Sea King was launched and it arrived over the ship just before 8 o'clock as the *Union Star* was among the breakers. The pilot, Lieutenant Commander Russell Smith, USN, made repeated attempts to lift the crew off. The winchman, Sub Lieutenant Stephen Marlow, was lowered to within fifteen feet of the deck with a swell of fifty feet, putting him in extreme danger, but he was unable to make contact with any of the crew.

At 8.15p.m., the *Solomon Browne* received the order to launch. In the crew were Nigel Brockman, aged forty-three, and his son Neil, aged seventeen. Coxswain Richards ordered Neil out: 'One member of each family is enough.'

The *Union Star* was now aground on the rocks and at 9.20p.m., the helicopter crew saw the lifeboat trying to run alongside it so that the crew could leave the deck house and run over the side and jump in. The helicopter crew looked on as the *Solomon Browne* was picked up by the waves and deposited on to the hatches of the coaster, then it slid off backwards into the sea. On the next run in, they saw people making a dash for the lifeboat and jumping in. Shortly afterwards a radio message was picked up from the lifeboat: 'To Falmouth from Penlee lifeboat – we have four off.'

Air/Sea Rescue: a Royal Navy helicopter about to lift Antonio Gioffredi and Patrizio Cozzi after their powerboat *Vaporella* overturned and sank in high seas during a powerboat race off the Channel Islands. Both men sustained serious injuries to their knees and chest in the 130 mph crash and were flown to hospital.

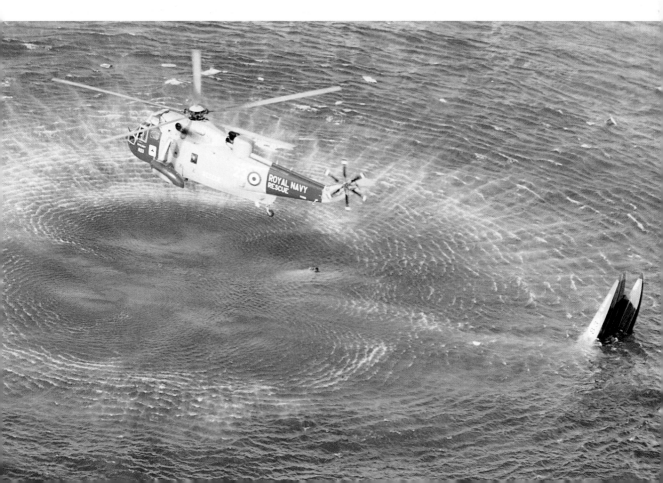

Unable to stay any longer, the helicopter moved away and returned to Culdrose, as Coxswain Richards turned to make another run past the *Union Star* which was now lying over on her side.

Nothing more was heard from the *Solomon Browne*. Captain Buurman called her several times but there was no reply. Relatives gathered on the quayside and round the coast, shining headlamps out to sea. At half past midnight, the St Mary's lifeboat was launched, but half an hour later the first pieces of wreckage were washed ashore at Lamorna Cove, unmistakably from the *Solomon Browne*; she had been smashed to pieces, possibly while making a last run alongside.

There were no survivors from the *Union Star* and all the *Solomon Browne*'s crew were lost, a devastating blow to the small community of Mousehole. Coxswain Trevelyan Richards was

The moment every rescue worker cherishes: a life saved against the odds, in this case a baby brought out alive from the devastation of the Mexico City earthquake in 1985.

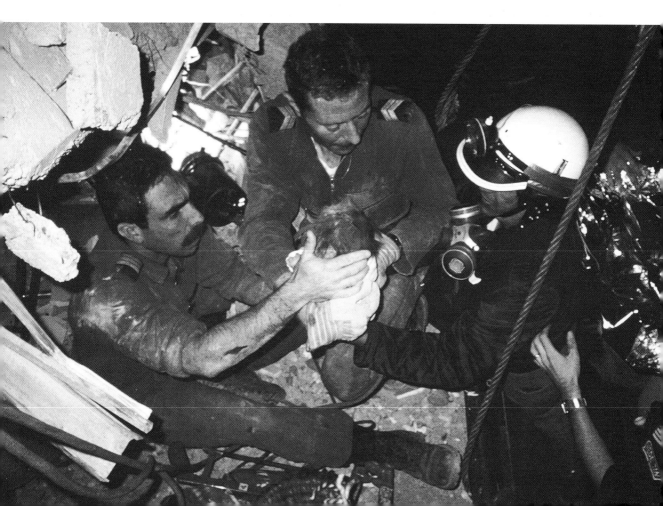

awarded the RNLI Gold Medal posthumously, and the whole crew was awarded the Bronze Medal. At the public inquiry, the chairman recorded that the loss of the *Solomon Browne* was due to 'persistent and heroic endeavours by the coxswain and his crew to save the lives of all from the *Union Star*. Such heroism enhances the highest traditions of the Royal National Lifeboat Institution in whose service they gave their lives.'

Examples of selfless, humanitarian action, especially those carried out with courage and coolness in the face of desperate circumstances, never fail to stir strong feelings of admiration and gratitude towards those special people in our society for they are a commonplace. They have given the Royal National Lifeboat Institution and its volunteer crews a very special place in British life, one which, after nearly two centuries, remains rooted in the people who serve in it. In November 1992, Neil Brockman, who had been left behind by Coxswain Richards that fateful night of the *Union Star* rescue, and whose father died on the *Solomon Browne*, became coxswain of the replacement Penlee lifeboat, the *Mabel Alice*.

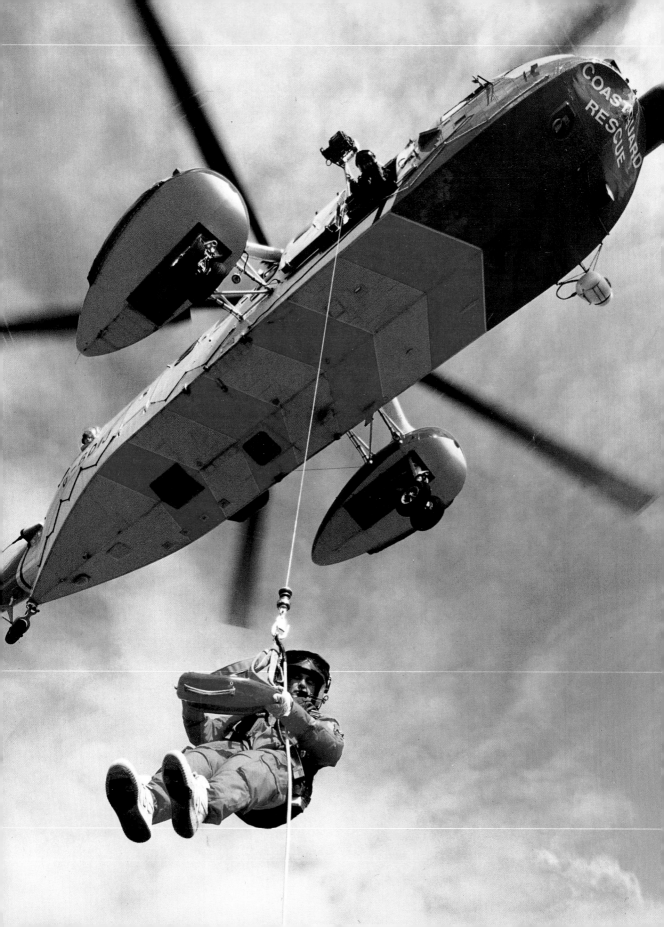

EPILOGUE

It is the nature of the modern media that headlines are made by the major natural and man-made disasters. Heart-warming stories of large numbers of people dramatically rescued or sombre accounts of tragic death when the efforts of the rescue services fail make the news and capture the imagination. These are occasions when the skill, training and dedication of the emergency services come together in moments of intense activity, but the daily round of routine work continues largely unrecorded and unremarked.

During filming for the second series of *Blues and Twos* there were many incidents which required courage, compassion and clear thinking, but which were unexceptional for members of the emergency services. Single stories from the filming are the most powerful testimony to their demanding, but largely unseen, everyday lives. A Thames Valley police officer was called to a house where, for several weeks, nothing had been heard of the old man who lived there. After hammering on the door first, she prepared to break it down, then heard a feeble response. The old man could not let her in because he had been unable to eat or get out of his armchair for three weeks. The officer waited until he struggled to the door, then arranged for him to be taken to hospital in an ambulance. Sadly he

Opposite: The coastguard has three Search and Rescue helicopters, two in Scotland, at Sumburgh in the Shetlands and at Stornaway in the Western Isles, and one at Lee-on-Solent on the south coast of England. The Lee-on-Solent aircraft featured in the first series of *Blues and Twos* rescuing twenty-two sailors from a tanker which was cut in two in a collision in the English Channel, and lifting a passenger who had had a heart attack on a cross-Channel ferry. The winchman is Tony Campbell.

215

died three weeks later. Fire fighters in Buckinghamshire brought a factory fire under control only to notice several pressurised acetylene bottles inside the smouldering building, still full of gas and heating up in the fire. With no more than a few words exchanged, they went in and hauled the bottles out, then dumped them in a skip filled with water to prevent them exploding. Ambulance workers, paramedics, casualty nurses and doctors in Edinburgh's Royal Infirmary at 3 o'clock in the morning on New Year's Day sorted out priorities for treatment from drunken and injured revellers in the crowded corridors.

Paramedics – who race to accidents by ambulance, on motor cycles, in four-wheel-drive jeeps or by helicopter – have a glamorous image, especially when they perform life-saving treatment for heart attacks on the pavement in central London. Such is the status of the paramedics today, that they have become fantasy figures. Many people dream of joining their ranks, but there are some, completely untrained individuals who have impersonated London Ambulance Service paramedics, listening for details on the rescue services' radio frequencies, then arriving at the scene dressed in green overalls with a first-aid bag and starting to treat the patient.

The reality of life as a paramedic is different: there is not much glamour in trying to decipher what a vomiting drug addict on the pavement is saying through the after-effects of an overdose.

The ability to show restraint under pressure and provocation is one of the key characteristics for serving in the modern emergency services. In Edinburgh, Derek Young and Steve Watkins went to treat a man who had been stabbed in the chest in a fight. He was bleeding as they put him in the ambulance, but most of his effort went into verbally abusing the men who were trying to help him, despite the endless calming and reassuring words from both of them that he would be all right. When his mother arrived she was ushered into the ambulance; the abuse continued until she clouted him, reminding him that he was speaking to ambulancemen, who she knew should be treated with respect.

Some people treat the ambulance service as a combination of Social Services, the Welfare State and the National Health Service on wheels. Most crew rooms have a fund of bizarre stories, such as the 999 call from a woman on a Friday night asking for a doctor to come to see her small son who had a temperature. On being told that it was not an emergency, and that it would be up to an hour before an ambulance could get to her, she cancelled the call because she was going out. Another tale involves a late-night call for an ambulance to take the morning-after pill to a woman who had just had unprotected sex with her boyfriend.

Both the television series and this book set out to show the kind of people who work in the emergency services – what they really do, how they do it, and how vital they are in a modern, civilised society. By showing people doing their everyday jobs, they should have shed a little more light on just how special these people are, and how fortunate we are to have such dedicated people in our emergency services. Nobody who has worked with them at the close quarters needed to make a series such as *Blues and Twos* would deny finding them very special indeed.

BIBLIOGRAPHY

In addition to many local, regional, national and overseas newspapers and periodicals, I have consulted the following books:

Gold Medal Rescues, Edward Wake-Walker, 1992.

A Century of Service to Mankind, A History of the St John Ambulance Brigade, Ronnie Cole-Mackintosh, 1986.

For Those in Peril, 50 Years of Royal Navy Search and Rescue, John Winton, 1992.

The Day of the Hillsborough Disaster, compiled by Rogan Taylor, Andrew Ward and Tim Newburn, 1995.

Piper Alpha, A Survivor's Story, Ed Punchard, 1989.

Zeebrugge, A Hero's Story, Stephen Ward, 1989.

Courage High! A History of Fire Fighting in London, Sally Holloway, 1992.

Fly for their Lives, John Chartres, 1988.

London's Armed Police, Robert W. Gould and Michael J. Waldren, 1986.

Hungerford, One Man's Massacre, Jeremy Josephs, 1993.

An Accident Waiting to Happen, Judith Cook, 1989.

The Accident and Crash Rescue Work of the Fire Service, Neil Wallington, 1987.

The Shell Book of Firsts, Patrick Robertson, 1974.

The Register of the George Cross, published by *This England*.